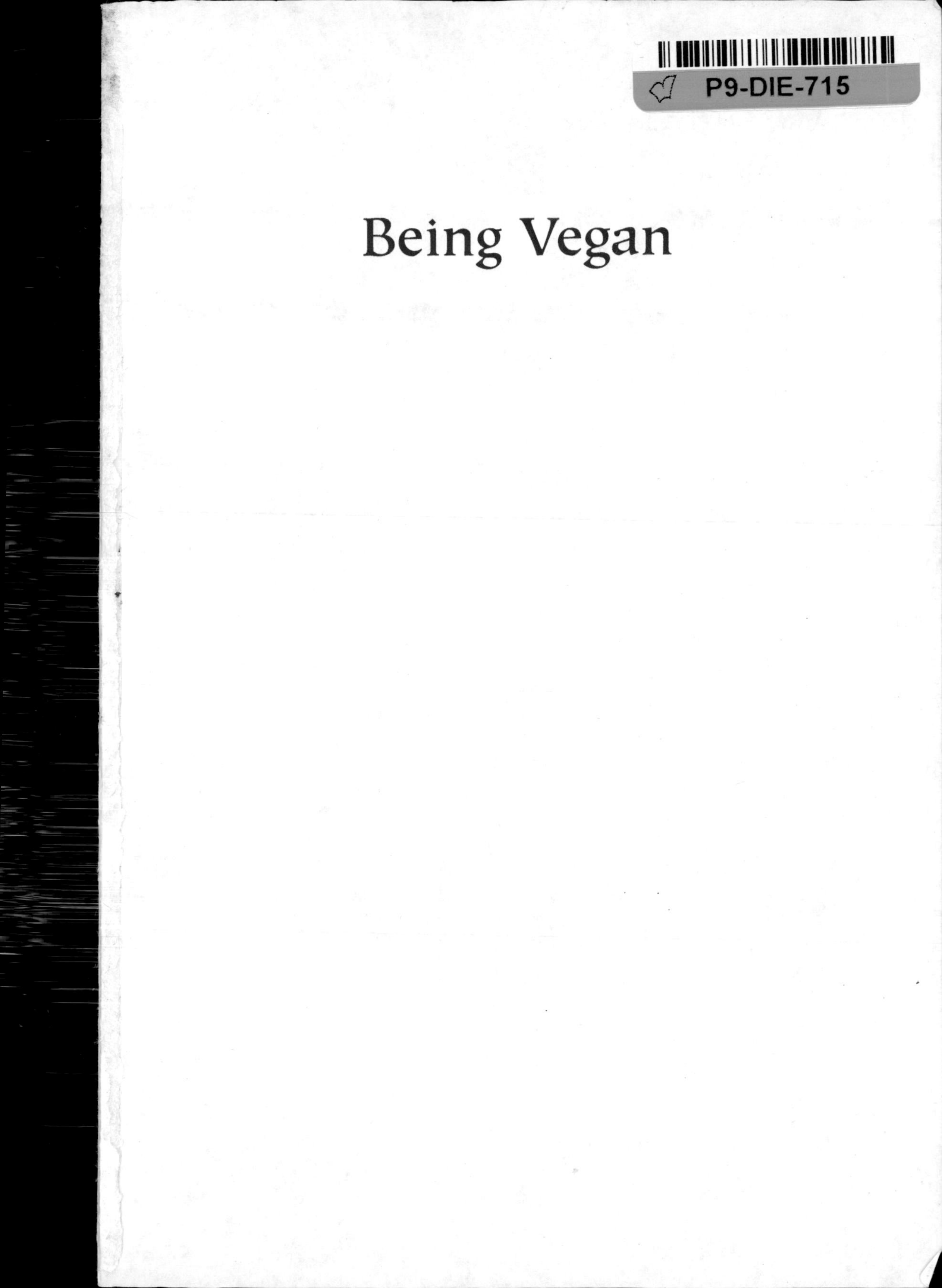

Being Vegan

Also by Joanne Stepaniak

The Vegan Sourcebook

The Saucy Vegetarian

Delicious Food for a Healthy Heart

Vegan Vittles

Table for Two

The Nutritional Yeast Cookbook

The Uncheese Cookbook

Ecological Cooking (with K. Hecker)

Vegan Deli

Being Vegan

Living with Conscience, Conviction, and Compassion

Joanne Stepaniak, M.S.Ed.

Foreword by Stanley M. Sapon, Ph.D.

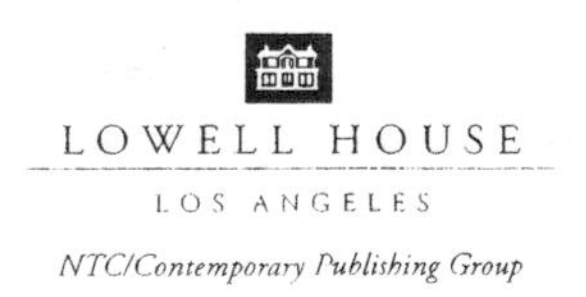

LOWELL HOUSE
LOS ANGELES
NTC/Contemporary Publishing Group

Library of Congress Cataloging-in-Publication Data

Stepaniak, Joanne, 1954-

Being vegan: living with conscience, conviction, and compassion / Joanne Stepaniak; foreword by Stanley M. Sapon.

p. cm.

Includes bibliographical references and index.

ISBN 0-7373-0323-9 (pbk.)

1. Veganism. I. Title.

TX392.S723 2000 00-042353

641.5'636–dc21

Published by Lowell House, a division of NTC/Contemporary Publishing Group, Inc.
4255 West Touhy Avenue, Lincolnwood, Illinois 60646-1975 U.S.A.

Managing Director and Publisher: Jack Artenstein
Executive Editor: Peter Hoffman
Director of Publishing Services: Rena Copperman
Managing Editor: Jama Carter
Project Editor: Claudia L. McCowan

Text Design: Kate Mueller
Cover illustration: Charlene Rendeiro © 2000

Printed and bound in the United States of America
International Standard Book Number: 1-7373-0323-9

6 7 8 9 0 DSH/DSH 0 1 0 9 8 7 6

This book is dedicated to all seekers of the compassionate way of life and to everyone who entrusted to me their questions and concerns about vegan living. I wish all of you goodness and peace as you travel the compassionate path.

Contents

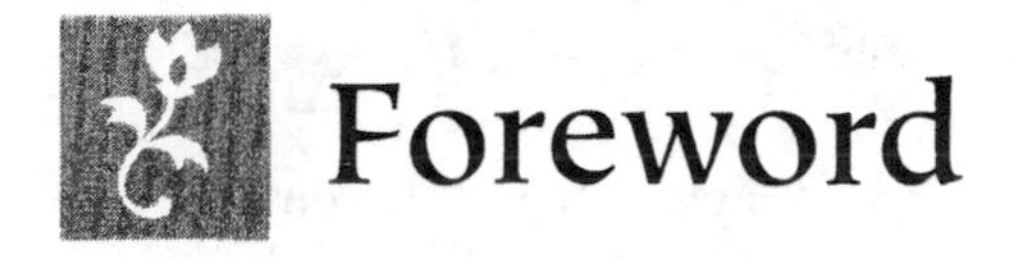

Foreword

When Joanne Stepaniak told me that she was writing a new book further exploring the themes of vegan philosophy, relationships, ethical practice, and food, I was delighted. Her work has always been distinguished by honest, courageous, and unclouded thought, penetrating behavioral insights, a soft wit, imaginative creativity, lucid writing, and a gift for guidance, in an all-encompassing grace and gentleness of spirit. Her writings are a source of illumination, information, inspiration, and empowerment for me and countless other readers. When she asked me to share some of my thoughts on vegan living in a foreword to the book, I felt both honored and privileged.

Humans have a unique and priceless capacity not only to assess and evaluate the consequences of their behavior, but the power to choose from a vast spectrum of existing alternatives, and even to create new ones. Distinguishing between kindness and cruelty is an exclusively human endeavor. And having invented this distinction, humans have gone on to declare the word *humane* to stand for the highest values of our species. The dictionary defines humane behavior as *characterized by kindness, mercy, or compassion,* indicating that kindness, mercy, and compassion are not one and the same.

Compassion describes what you *feel.* Kindness and mercy characterize what you *do.* Mercy can be seen as compassion in action. Comparatively speaking, it is easier to acknowledge the respect due another living creature than it is to put that respect into action.

Although we may now be thoughtful adults daring to live by an unconventional set of ethical values, most of us are still burdened by the baggage of a shared behavioral and cultural history. We have been reared (and continue to live) in a cultural environment that socializes children according to a set of unwritten and unspoken—but strictly enforced—protocols for exhibiting compassionate, merciful behavior.

It is obvious that children are taught—most insistently—to feel compassion for their families, their friends, adherents of their faith, their countrypeople. What is not so apparent is that children are also painstakingly taught what society considers the appropriate limit to the display of compassion—*where to draw the line,* at what point we must put a stop to the growing circles of compassion. Our culture even goes on to designate those people whose misfortunes we may applaud and those people whom we may be prompted to harm.

It is one thing to acknowledge the heightened awareness that leads to the decision to adopt a vegan lifestyle. Implementing that decision and making its underlying principles a working part of our everyday living involves benefits and costs. The benefits are deep personal satisfaction and inner harmony. But there is a cost to caring. When we vow to respect the integrity of another creature's life, we oblige ourselves to surrender the profit, pleasure, or convenience we have enjoyed from the exploitation of that being—animal or human.

Part of the wizardry of Joanne's work is found in the gentleness with which she cultivates and nurtures the spirit of compassion in her audience, and the wisdom and integrity of her counsel in easing and facilitating the merciful behavior that compassion calls for. The outcome of her efforts dependably leads us all a step forward in experiencing the joys of vegan living.

If we would live in ways that diminish conflict, violence, pain, and suffering in the world, we can make no better or more productive effort than to cultivate our awareness of the feelings of other sentient creatures, and strive to extend to all of them precisely the kind of benevolent mercy we ask for ourselves. How can we accomplish this? Ask Joanne!

—STANLEY M. SAPON, PH.D.
Emeritus Professor of Psycholinguistics, University of Rochester
Co-founder, The Maimonides Project

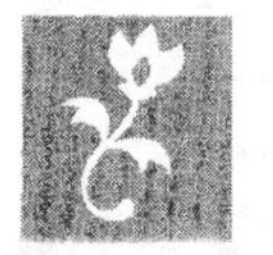

Prologue

This book is a distillation and compilation of some of the thousands of questions I have received about compassionate vegan living through my Web site, Grassroots Veganism; award-winning on-line advice column, Ask Joanne!; and the print version of this column, which appears quarterly in *Vegetarian Voice* magazine, a publication of the North American Vegetarian Society. People from every corner of the world have contacted me, including those who reside in remote regions where it would seem nearly impossible to know about vegans, let alone be one. I have also heard from individuals all across the United States and Canada, spanning the continuum from teenagers to college students to grandparents, from progressive urban centers to loose-knit suburban communities to isolated rural towns. This has made me steadfastly aware that vegans comprise a heterogeneous population hailing from every age group, income level, ethnicity, and race. Together we present a vibrant and diverse perspective on a multitude of issues from politics to childrearing to spirituality. There is no single representative vegan voice. We are many voices, many cultures, and many spirits melding into one.

Frequently I receive similar questions from numerous people living thousands of miles apart or even on separate continents. This demonstrates that despite our divergent backgrounds, vegans share common interests and collective concerns. We want to have a clear understanding of the philosophy and ethics that form the foundation of our lifestyle and guide our daily decisions. We want to figure out how to put these values into practical service in our day-to-day lives. And we all want to bring the fruits of our compassion into our relationships and onto our tables.

Just when I think I've heard every inquiry imaginable, questions emerge about topics and situations I had not previously contemplated, and I am yet again astounded by the depth of consideration vegans bring to their choices. The profound caring that vegans demonstrate is nothing short of awe-inspiring. Regardless of our demographics, vegans are unified through a shared belief in universal compassion and an unwavering commitment to peace, nonviolence, and justice for all people, animals, and the earth. Responding to their queries is an incredible honor and a responsibility that I take quite seriously. I trust that the questions and answers contained in this book will foster a greater appreciation for and understanding of veganism as well as offer hope, support, insight, and encouragement to those who seek a more compassionate way of life.

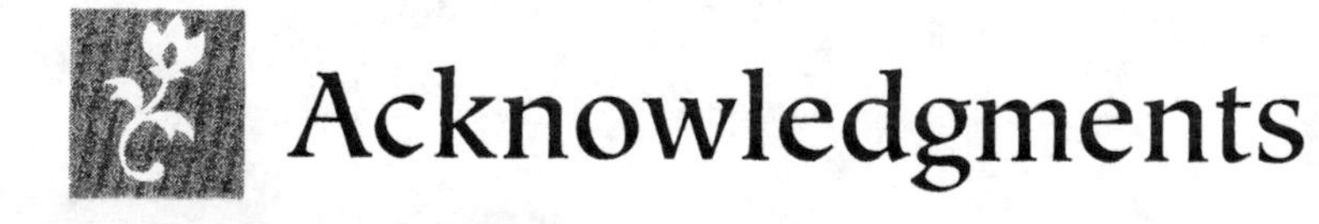

Acknowledgments

My deepest gratitude is extended to Jeff and Sabrina Nelson, the incomparable founders of VegSource, without whose generosity this book would not have been possible; to Peggy Burris, who epitomizes the meaning of altruism and friendship; to Stan and Rhoda Sapon for their unflagging support and loving-kindness; and to my beloved Michael, as always. Special appreciation is also extended to my editor, Hudson Perigo, for her skillful guidance and exceptional insights.

May peace and joy be yours.

Chapter 1

Vegan Philosophy

Putting Down Roots

To understand what it means to be vegan, it is vital to reflect on the historical roots and origin of the word. Many people think of the term *vegan* and its associated lifestyle as something new or insurgent. In many ways, just the opposite is true.

The word *vegan* was coined by Donald Watson in 1944 in Leicester, England. He, along with several other members of the Vegetarian Society, wanted to form an alliance of nondairy vegetarians as a subgroup of the Society. When their proposal was rejected, they ventured to start their own organization. They considered what to call themselves, and, after evaluating a range of ingenious possibilities, agreed that vegan (decisively pronounced VEE-gn, with a long "e" and hard "g") was best. It was derived from the word *vegetarian* by taking the first three letters (veg) and the last two letters (an) because, as Donald Watson explained, "veganism starts with vegetarianism and carries it through to its logical conclusion."

In late 1944, The Vegan Society was established, advocating a totally plant-based diet excluding flesh, fish, fowl, eggs, honey, and animals' milk, butter, and cheese, and also encouraging the manufacture and use of alternatives to animal commodities, including clothing and shoes. The group argued that the elimination of exploitation of any kind was necessary to achieve a more reasonable and humane society. From its inception, veganism was defined as a philosophy and way of living. It was never intended to be merely a diet. *Vegan* still today describes a lifestyle and belief system that revolves around a reverence for life.

In 1960, the American Vegan Society was founded by Jay Dinshah. It embraced the principles of its British predecessor, advocating a strictly plant-based diet and a lifestyle free of animal products. In addition, the American Vegan Society championed the philosophy of *ahimsa,* a Sanskrit word interpreted as "dynamic harmlessness," along with encouraging service to humanity, nature, and creation. In other words, in order to practice veganism, it is not sufficient to simply avoid specific foods and products; it is necessary to actively participate in beneficial selfless action as well.

Omitting animal products from one's life is a passive action; it does not require asserting oneself, it merely involves avoidance. To implement *ahimsa,* we must engage the dynamic part of "dynamic harmlessness." Therefore, to fully apply the vegan ethic, not only are vegans compelled to do the least harm, they are obliged to do the most good.

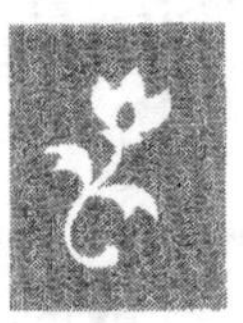

Veganism is not merely passive resistance. It compels practitioners to make deliberate and dynamic choices about each and every activity in their lives and to consider the impact and benefit of their actions.

Being vegan is at once complex, challenging, and rewarding because each element of a vegan's life is chosen with conscious awareness. When people decide to be vegan, they make an ethical commitment to bettering themselves and the world around them. This pledge is not to be taken lightly. It requires us to seriously examine all facets of our lives. When we delve more deeply into its essence, we see that a vegan outlook extends far beyond the material and tangible. Vegan perspectives permeate our relationships, spiritual beliefs, occupations, and pastimes. Indeed, there are few areas of life that the vegan ethic doesn't touch or influence to one degree or another.

Becoming vegan is a process; rarely does someone convert to complete veganism overnight. More typically, people transition to a vegan lifestyle, generally altering their diet first and then gradually replacing their clothing, cosmetics, and incongruous habits with more serene, compassionate options. In truth, there is no end to the vegan journey. We are perpetually challenged to do more, to strive higher, to see and understand more clearly, to be more loving and humble. This is the gift of veganism. It is a guide for compassionate living. It is the path of honoring our roots, our planet, all life, and ourselves.

It is necessary to understand the principles that frame vegan practice in order to apply them to our lives. In its Articles of Association, The Vegan Society in England defines veganism as follows:

> Veganism denotes a philosophy and way of living which seeks to exclude—as far as is possible and practical—all forms of exploitation of, and cruelty to, animals for food, clothing, or any other purpose; and by extension, promotes the development and use of animal-free alternatives for the benefit of humans, animals, and the environment.

As a guide for vegan living, the American Vegan Society delineates six pillars of the compassionate way. Combining the first letter of each pillar spells out the word *ahimsa,* the philosophy of nonviolence practiced and promoted by Mahatma Gandhi.

1. Abstinence from animal products
2. Harmlessness with reverence for life
3. Integrity of thought, word, and deed
4. Mastery over oneself
5. Service to humanity, nature, and creation
6. Advancement of understanding and truth

Based on these explanations, the practice of veganism entails abstaining from the use of animal products in every aspect of daily living *as much as is possible and practical.* Although this includes what one eats, it also extends to all other types of consumables. In addition, vegan practice is coupled with the active pursuit of alternatives to commodities typically made from or with animal products or by-products, as well as the avoidance of animal exploitation and cruelty *for any purpose.* Therefore, veganism is not merely passive resistance. It compels practitioners to make deliberate choices about every activity in their lives and to consider the impact and benefit of their actions.

Although the basic tenets of veganism are fairly straightforward, there are many circumstances we encounter for which an ethical vegan option appears ambiguous–times when determining what is possible and what is practical becomes convoluted. In our modern world, where nearly everything is contaminated with minute amounts of animal derivatives and many of our principled choices turn out to be paradoxical, we must concede that it is virtually impossible to maintain absolute vegan compliance. Consequently, vegans occasionally need clarification on particular issues, seek help determining the most humane choices, or want assistance when they become preoccupied with the impractical.

This chapter tackles some of the hidden and not-so-hidden philosophical quandaries that confront vegans from time to time. By shedding a little light on the nuances of vegan precepts we can unravel some of the confusion that sometimes surrounds them.

Definitions and Delineations

Can you tell me all the kinds of vegans there are?

Vegans are big, small, old, young, tall, short, gay, straight, thin, fat, single, married, wealthy, poor, Asian, black, Hispanic, white, brown, "green," Jewish, Christian, Hindu, Buddhist, Jain, Muslim, agnostic, atheist, Democrat, Republican, socialist, capitalist, leftist, rightist, liberal, conservative–well, you get the picture.

The term *vegetarian* was created in 1847 by the people who eventually became the first members of the Vegetarian Society of Great Britain. It refers to individuals who do not eat meat, fowl, or fish. The word *vegetarian* encompasses strictly what one eats and does not allude to any other behavior. As a result, there are many different kinds of vegetarians because there is a wide range of food choices within these parameters. There are vegetarians who are ovo, lacto, ovolacto, macrobiotic, fruitarian, raw foodist, natural hygiene, oil-free, fat-free, sugar-free, high-protein, low-carbohydrate, and so on. Within the boundaries of the basic definition, the possibilities are limitless. This is because there is no ideology behind the meaning of vegetarian that consolidates each person's individual perspective or motivation.

Therefore, people may choose to be vegetarian for any number of reasons and their diets may differ vastly. Because vegetarianism deals exclusively with food, the concept of a "vegetarian lifestyle" is basically an oxymoron. The only thing one vegetarian has in common with any other vegetarian is what he doesn't eat.

Contrary to vegetarianism, veganism was founded on deeply held ethical convictions that espouse a dynamic respect for all life. This philosophy unifies vegans everywhere, regardless of superficial differences. Thus a vegan from one part of the world can relate to and empathize with a vegan from another part of the world despite their disparate cultures and languages.

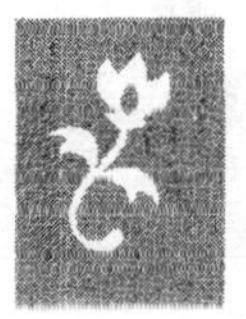

Veganism is more than what a person does or doesn't *eat*—it comprises who a person *is*.

There are no such entities as "part-time vegans," "partial vegans," or "dietary vegans." People who just have a plant-based diet are not vegans; they are *total vegetarians*. Until one's commitment extends beyond the scope of food, the word *vegan* does not apply, regardless of how the media or certain individuals or groups wish to employ it. Unlike vegetarianism, being vegan does not entail simply what a person does or doesn't *eat*–it comprises who a person *is*.

People who are vegan attempt to imbue every aspect of their lives with an ethic of compassion. This influences their day-to-day choices and colors their political perspectives, social attitudes, and personal relationships. This is not to say that all vegans think alike, act the same, or view the world and their place in it identically. Nevertheless, vegans do subscribe to a shared tenet that builds a collective awareness. It is this coalescence of consciousness that creates a bond among vegans and has the power to transcend cursory distinctions. In the final analysis, despite our diversity, there is only one type of vegan–a person who is committed to and practices reverence and respect for all life.

Is veganism just an animal rights adjunct? If not, to what extent is it a life philosophy or theology such as stoicism or Taoism?

Veganism is not directly related to animal rights, although it makes sense for animal rights activists to practice a vegan lifestyle. Eating, wearing, or using products derived from animals while defending the rights of other animals is contradictory behavior known as *selective compassion*. Consequently, many animal rights campaigners are vegans, but social or political activism is not fundamental to veganism.

Veganism is a philosophy that espouses reverence for life. It is not a theology and does not contemplate religious truth. Its tenets are relatively simple–in a nutshell, do the least harm and the most good–but their application can at times seem complex. Veganism does not demand prohibitions to transform practitioners' outlook or character. Just the opposite is true. People are drawn to veganism because they already acknowledge the inherent value in all living beings. Vegan ideology is a guide for how to put these personal convictions into action and apply them realistically to daily life.

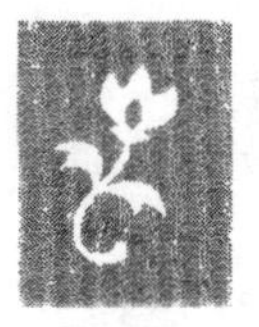

Vegan tenets are relatively simple: Do the least harm and the most good.

What about human animals?

Because vegan principles honor all living beings, our fellow humans must be equally respected and embraced, even though sometimes this can be one of the most difficult aspects of vegan practice. Often it is necessary to work on our own issues instead of attempting to change the people we dislike or don't get along with. This includes how we handle conflict and criticism and deal with our own feelings of anger. In each challenging human interaction, we must ask ourselves: How can I avoid doing harm to myself or to others? How can I help improve the situation?

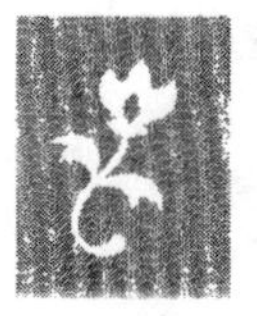

The vegan concepts of *ahimsa* and dynamic harmlessness extend to people no less than to other animals.

Veganism, in all its simplicity, provides a highly sophisticated path for personal development and inner growth. It summons us to explore our deepest resources and concede our strengths and weaknesses. A vegan lifestyle is not for the faint of heart nor slight of spirit. It requires courage, dedication, and willingness to dig deep inside to discover our greatest promise. It allows us to effect the positive changes we yearn for by actively implementing them and by being an abiding example of the peaceful world we envision.

Can I call myself vegan if I still use, eat, or wear a few products that contain animal-derived ingredients?

According to the most concise definitions set forth by The Vegan Society (England), the American Vegan Society, and the Oxford English Dictionaries, the word *vegan* refers to "a person who does not eat or use animal products." Therefore, using, ingesting, or wearing products derived from animals does not comply with the accepted definition of vegan.

Nevertheless, animal by-products are so pervasive that it is sometimes impossible to avoid them. In addition, vegan alternatives are not yet obtainable for all animal-based commodities, so vegans must, by necessity, make a few concessions.

If vegans focus on the larger picture and avoid the obvious animal products and by-products, then being vegan becomes much more practical and attainable. There are hardly any food or clothing items for which a vegan needs to compromise, because convenient substitutes are readily available. When there are no vegan possibilities at hand, most vegans can simply do without. Making nonvegan choices when animal-free options exist is not vegan.

An individual can still practice the central tenets of veganism even though basic compliance has not yet been met. However, technically speaking, this person would not be vegan. She or he might be "transitioning to veganism" or be a "total vegetarian." Because *vegan* is a descriptive term that is neither favorable nor pejorative, interpreting *vegan* as positive or negative is a personal judgment. The word itself is neutral.

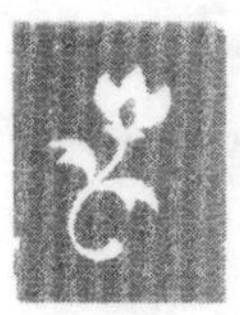

Vegan is not a rank nor a badge of excellence. It is merely a word that describes individuals who are distinctly committed to revering all life by conforming to a clearly delineated code of ethical behavior.

Some people who aspire to be vegan or vegetarian label themselves as such even though they do not explicitly observe the principal criteria of these practices. Take, for instance, the chicken-eating, fish-eating, just-no-red-meat-eating "vegetarian." Regrettably, this has created confusion regarding the definition of vegetarian and has led to misuse of the word by the media, health care practitioners, and the public. Such deviation renders the term meaningless.

Vegan is not a rank nor a badge of excellence. It is merely a word that describes individuals who are distinctly committed to revering all life by conforming to a clearly delineated code of ethical behavior. Its significance lies in its accuracy. Describing oneself as vegan while continuing to use products that are conspicuously animal-based could easily contribute to the corruption of the term.

I do not eat any animal products for both health and ethical reasons, but I am not a true vegan because I wear leather shoes and wool suits. However, I have found that it's helpful to use the term *vegan* to describe my diet, especially in restaurants, to make it clear to most people what I do not eat. Is this appropriate?

It is understandable that someone who is a total vegetarian but not a vegan would want to use the word *vegan* in a restaurant to get the point across. It's clear, concise, and it works. *Total vegetarian* might work, too, as could *strict vegetarian,* with a simple explanation of what is and isn't acceptable. (People often have to do that when using the term *vegan* anyway.) But being vegan is more than the sum of what one does and doesn't eat. It also goes beyond personal health motivations. Many people who eventually become ethical vegans initially are drawn to an animal-free diet because of health concerns and then adopt additional rationales as they learn about new issues. In fact, health is probably the prime motivator for most people to move toward a more plant-centered diet.

As a comparison, there are also people who believe that kosher food is "cleaner" and more healthful than nonkosher food. For observant Jews, keeping kosher is a component of their Judaism. However, non-Jews who keep kosher are not deemed Jewish simply because they follow a kosher diet. There is a gulf of difference between the lifestyle, motivation, and commitment of the observant Jew and the person who just wants to eat like one.

Labels can be valuable designations for clarity. When used as such, they do not condemn or condone individual choices; instead, they elucidate, identify, and describe.

I want to help preserve the meaning of the words *vegan* and *vegetarian.* It upsets me to see people who call themselves vegetarian when they eat fish or chicken. It makes it confusing for the world at large because the public gets the wrong idea of what vegetarians eat. As for vegan, it is my understanding that there can be both ethical vegans and dietary vegans. Is this right?

To understand the difference between the words *vegetarian* and *vegan,* and to appreciate their full meaning, it is important to investigate their histories. The term *vegetarian* was devised solely to describe diet—nothing else. On the other hand, the term *vegan* encompasses far more than just what one eats. It is—and has always been—a philosophy of compassionate living, and this is a vital distinction.

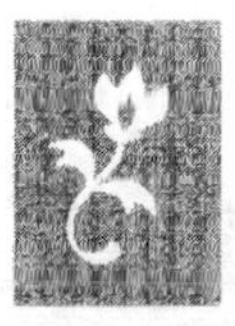

Vegetarianism deals only with food, but food is just one aspect of being vegan.

Despite what many U.S. dictionaries state, to define vegan otherwise is inaccurate. Even in England, where the term was introduced, it still took the Oxford English Dictionary well over two decades to finally describe it correctly. Probably this was because it was so difficult for anyone to understand the concept of living—not just eating—without animal products. Some U.S. dictionaries even list alternative pronunciations (such as VAY-gn or VEJ-n), which are blatantly wrong according to both The Vegan Society (in England) and the American Vegan Society, our founding organization in the United States. Donald Watson, who coined the term, was adamant about the word's pronunciation and meaning. That's why it's up to those who practice a vegan lifestyle and those who are affiliated with vegans to set the record straight, and, hopefully, one day our dictionaries will get the message, too.

"Dietary vegan" is one way to get around the sticky issue of those who consume no animal products but do not extend the animal-free philosophy beyond diet, but I'm not sure it is the best choice. In a way, this is like using the term "secular Catholic" for people who want to pick and choose which aspects of Catholicism they want to practice. Catholic is Catholic and vegan is vegan. To put a qualifier before either of these words dilutes their meaning, detracts from those who actually practice these lifestyles, and confounds the media. This is what happened with the term *vegetarian,* and now doing damage control is practically impossible. Today there is a whole slew of people who truly believe "Of course vegetarians eat fish and chicken—who are *you* to say they don't?" A similar distortion could easily occur with the word *vegan.*

For us to prevent this from happening, it is crucial that vegans educate themselves and their friends and families, the media, and the public, to maintain control of the original meaning and purpose of these words. The expressions "total vegetarian," "pure vegetarian," and "strict vegetarian" are more applicable to people who are "dietary vegans," and they have been used effectively for decades. They are more germane because vegetarian has always dealt only with food, but food is only one aspect of being vegan. Another way to characterize people who are not yet vegan but are headed in that direction is "transitioning to veganism."

Although this matter may be relatively minor in light of the broader purpose of humane living, insisting on the accurate usage of our defining terminology is critical to prevent *vegan* from heading down the same slippery slope as *vegetarian.*

I am fourteen and in the process of becoming a vegan. I have read that to be a full vegan you must perform charitable acts and things along that line. I believe that I am not old enough to participate in activities like protests. I do, however, have three dogs and a cat, all of whom we took in from rescue societies and the streets. My mother and I always stop to take in stray animals and try to find them homes. Is this enough to contribute to the vegan cause?

Vegan living involves doing the least harm and the most good. This applies to all situations and extends to human relationships as well. "Charitable acts" simply refers to being kind, thoughtful, and compassionate toward the earth and all life. It does not mean that vegans must participate in protests or any other specific action. In fact, sometimes protests result in anger, abusive language, or behavior that is harmful to others or oneself. Such scenarios can be counterproductive and are not necessarily representative of the vegan approach or philosophy.

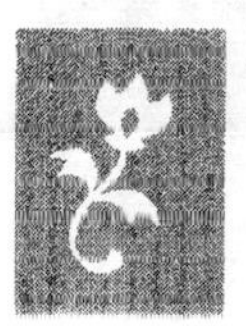

Each moment of our lives we have the option to do right, do wrong, or do nothing. Attempting to do right as often as we can is all that being vegan requires.

People who are old enough to make decisions about their life—for instance, what to eat, what to wear, what to say, or whom to choose as friends—can behave in a veganly fashion. Regardless of age, we all make choices every day that can affect others in a positive or negative way. Philosophic veganism guides practitioners to opt for alternatives that bring joy, peace, comfort, and harmony whenever possible. Small acts of consideration, generosity, and respect—such as helping your brother or sister with homework, taking the dog for a walk, visiting a sick friend, washing the dishes after dinner, cleaning the cat's litter box, doing the laundry, showing gratitude, or straightening your room—are all part of vegan behavior. In addition, veganism encourages compassionate feelings including forgiveness, selflessness, and empathy, which can lead to compassionate deeds. It also supports self-growth in ways that inspire inner and outer peace. Therefore, some vegans are motivated to learn to play a musical instrument or sing; others pursue training in conflict resolution; and still others are prompted to plant a garden, study dance, or learn to cook. There are endless ways to perform "charitable acts," and there are probably many ways in which you already engage in vegan activities without even acknowledging them as such.

Adopting animals in need and finding loving homes for strays is an exemplary act of altruism. There is no reason to keep score and tally your good deeds each day to measure up to some arbitrary number that would qualify you for vegan status. No such number exists. Most people know in their heart what is right behavior, but we often elect to go a different route because other choices are easier, more familiar, or more comfortable.

Each moment of our lives we have the option to do right, do wrong, or do nothing. Attempting to do right as often as we can is all that being vegan requires.

Theology and Spirituality

I researched the word *ahimsa,* and I feel that I understand it. But what is the vegan belief regarding our beginning, the Creator, and evolution?

Veganism is a philosophy of life; it is not a religion. Nevertheless, many practitioners find the vegan ethic provides them with a moral beacon akin to most religious precepts. This is because vegan principles influence nearly every aspect of daily living in very constructive and pragmatic ways.

The tenets of veganism are guideposts for how we should live our life. They do not postulate on how life began or evolved and do not dictate nonsecular concepts or beliefs. Vegans are free to follow any spiritual path they desire, and any person committed to a particular religious perspective should find no conflict in practicing a vegan lifestyle.

Are Christianity and veganism compatible?

Although veganism is not a religion, many people find moral guidance and spiritual solace in the vegan ethic. Because vegan principles are so all-encompassing, they often function as a core value system for practitioners.

Vegans come from all walks of life as well as all religious affiliations and spiritual perspectives. There are numerous biblical passages that support a cruelty-free lifestyle. Nevertheless, when opposing groups engage in scriptural sparring, they each invariably unearth every imaginable excerpt to support their contrary positions.

A person may believe in a Supreme Being or higher power who created all life. It would certainly take a cruel deity to beget sentient beings whose sole purpose is to suffer and die at the hands of humans. One argument opposed to a vegan lifestyle is that Christianity contends that nonhuman animals do not have souls and therefore cannot go to heaven. If one believes this, then it makes even more sense that we be as kind as possible to animals now, since this is the only life they may experience.

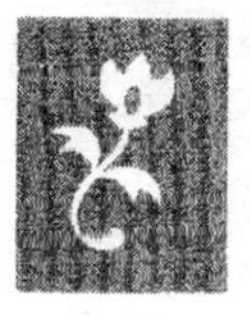

Vegan practice is the dynamic embodiment of the most celebrated religious ideals.

Judeo-Christian theology embraces the Ten Commandments, the precepts given to Moses on Mount Sinai. The commandment "Thou shalt not kill" is a tenet that the people of Israel and their followers—including Jesus and his followers—were mandated to obey. Vegan principles exemplify this directive. Furthermore, those who practice vegan living and believe in a higher power can honor their god more fully by actively protecting and defending all life and all creation.

None of the world's major religions assert that "might makes right." However, when we take the lives of other animals in the name of food or clothing, we are contending just that. Killing other animals becomes even more heinous in light of the fact that we have innumerable alternatives to animal products for virtually every commodity.

Veganism is compatible with Christianity and essentially all other major religions. In fact, it could very well be said that vegan practice is the dynamic embodiment of the most celebrated religious ideals.

I am a vegetarian and want to know why, in the Bible, God tells people to make animal sacrifices and that animals are for them to eat.

One of the earliest passages in the Bible that censures the eating of animal flesh is the following excerpt from Genesis 1:29:

> And God said, Behold, I have given you every herb bearing seed, which is upon the face of all the earth, and every tree, in which is the fruit of a tree yielding seed; to you it shall be for meat.

Although some biblical selections appear to contradict this admonition, numerous other passages support it.

There are many ways to interpret biblical text, depending on your individual religious views. Some Christian sects believe the Bible is the exact word of God; therefore, it must be followed to the letter. But many other denominations construe the Bible in terms of its historical context and rich symbolism. They acknowledge that much biblical language does not translate effectively into contemporary vernacular and therefore cannot not be fully understood in terms of our modern cultural perspectives.

Even for those who believe that God instructed humans to have "dominion" over other animals, dominion should be understood as benevolent guardianship, not domination. If people loved animals the way God loved them in the Garden of Eden, we would never consider using them for selfish gratification and power. As the Bible explains, God cherishes all creation. Those who respect the rights and lives of animals by not eating them, killing them, or using them for self-serving purposes are following the path back to Eden–a path reflective of God's love and compassion for all life.

Personal Well-Being and Diet

I have a friend who has been a strict vegan for about three years. My concern is that she has a number of serious medical conditions. However, she adamantly refuses even to consult with a physician because she is certain that all medications contain animal products or have been tested on animals. When I try to counsel a sense of proportion and urge her at least to consider where her vegan morals conflict with the principle of self-preservation, she accuses me of being a shameless apologist and is horrified that I would suggest she compromise her beliefs. Help!

Vegans and nonvegans alike often consider compassion in terms of others, rarely applying a similar standard of caring to themselves. It is as though we feel unworthy of the kindness we give away or believe that benevolence toward oneself is a selfish indulgence. According to Western perspectives, altruism, by its very nature, is other-directed.

This viewpoint, however, is extremely narrow in scope. Without respect and love for oneself, how can a person ever truly understand what it means to give and receive on any meaningful level? Compassion begins with nurturing the self. Jumping into external forms of empathy while bypassing one's own needs is akin to running without first learning how to walk.

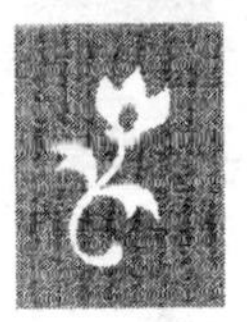

If compassion is the heart of vegan practice,
then caring for oneself is the heart of compassion.

If your friend has serious maladies, they need to be addressed as soon as possible by a physician or other health professional. Some people use veganism as an easy way to bypass an examination or doctor's visit and abstain from taking medication. However, being vegan does not absolve practitioners from taking personal responsibility for their physical and mental well-being.

If compassion is the heart of vegan practice, then caring for oneself is the heart of compassion. When no other options exist, vegans are obliged to do whatever is necessary to sustain their health because our own life and vitality are certainly not worth less than anyone else's. Sometimes this entails small compromises for the short run, but this in no way forestalls the higher objectives of veganism. Harming ourselves by abstaining from appropriate care does more to negate vegan practice than making minor concessions. Not taking care of oneself is not fully practicing compassion, which in turn means not truly honoring the aim of vegan principles.

Is it better to not take prescription drugs that have been tested on animals so you don't support the vivisection industry, or to take them so the animals didn't die in vain?

Many people falsely assume that when pharmaceutical products are tested on animals, it is a single animal that suffers and dies. In reality, countless lives are sacrificed each time a new drug enters the marketplace. There is no way to pay homage to the animals that are needlessly obliterated for research. Utilizing products whose manufacture involved animal testing does not honor these animals or vindicate their vivisectors. Because the Food and Drug Administration (FDA) mandates animal testing for each pharmaceutical drug or compound, all prescription medications are subject to this process.

The vegan ethic does not require people to perform deeds of heroic proportions. Therefore, if vegans are prescribed a drug for their physical or mental well-being, vegan principles would not preclude them from taking it. There is no way to rekindle the lives of those animals that died during pharmaceutical research, so boycotting vital life- or health-saving products because they were tested on animals would be foolish.

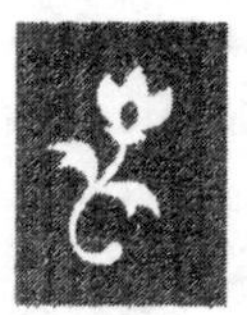

The vegan ethic does not require people to perform deeds of heroic proportions.

However, vegans can and should support the implementation of humane alternatives to vivisection, so that this moral conflict will cease to exist. In the meantime, vegans in need of medications should not eschew them nor allow themselves to feel guilty or culpable for doing what is necessary to maintain their health or their lives.

I am thinking about becoming a vegan. I have really bad allergies to milk and some other foods. I have read that a vegan diet can make some allergies better, but I am afraid that this would seem weird to my family and friends.

It sounds as though you are contemplating adopting a total vegetarian diet, not necessarily a vegan lifestyle, because of concerns about your allergies and health. It is important to acknowledge the difference between an animal-free diet and a compassionate lifestyle, because one is rooted in the head and the other in the heart.

When people make dietary changes based on theories about what is best for their health, there is no impetus to maintain the diet if their health declines or their hypotheses prove false. Tinkering with what we eat or don't eat to determine what makes us feel better doesn't involve an ethical commitment. It is a choice that has the potential to change in an instant, especially if opposing medical concepts surface. True veganism, however, is a lifestyle—not merely a diet—based on the moral conviction that all living beings are sacred.

Our culture finds it easier to accept dietary deviations due to health-related matters than preferences based on principle. There is no need to argue for a way of eating that reverses the progression of a disease, prevents an allergic reaction, facilitates weight loss, reduces our cholesterol level, improves the condition of our skin, or enhances our overall sense of physical well-being. Who would contest this? Where is the controversy? No caring person would insist that we return to a meat-based diet if it would impair our health. Meat-eaters might say they feel sorry for us, but they would not condemn us.

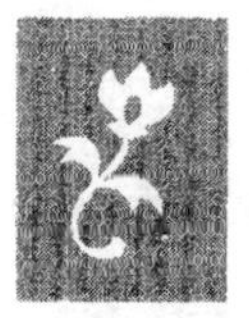

An animal-free diet is rooted in the head.
A compassionate lifestyle is rooted in the heart.

Alternatively, modern society views moral precepts as elective and therefore capable of being modified or discarded whenever they are inconvenient, disruptive, or unsettling to others. In fact, our culture sees this as not only reasonable but necessary for individuals to function as part of the greater whole. As a result, people who choose a principled lifestyle are often forced to defend their beliefs and practices to those who see their tenets as optional, not imperative.

To be considered weird because one aspect of your life—your diet—alleviates a health condition is deemed defensible. To be labeled peculiar because of who you *are* and what you *assert* is another matter altogether and one that is much more difficult to endure.

Your family and friends do not want you to endanger your health, regardless of whether or not they choose to continue to eat meat. Try a plant-based diet. If it makes you feel better and eliminates your allergies, your glowing vitality will be argument enough to support your choice.

I am recovering from an eating disorder. Now that I am healthy, I feel I can honestly look at the ethical reasons why I want to become vegan. However, during my hospitalizations I noticed that many women with anorexia were also vegetarian or vegan. By the end of their treatment, most were eating meat again (not me, of course). What is your opinion on the connection, if any, between vegetarianism or veganism and eating disorders?

There is absolutely no relationship between veganism and eating disorders. Veganism is a compassionate way of life; anorexia nervosa is a debilitating psychological and endocrine disorder characterized by a pathological fear of gaining weight. People with anorexia nervosa develop faulty eating habits that typically lead to malnutrition and excessive weight loss.

Unfortunately, some anorexics use vegetarianism and veganism as a shield for their inadequate eating patterns and an excuse for avoiding food. This has led to an erroneous association between veganism and anorexia and has caused confusion among health professionals, the media, and the public. This spurious link has generated a slew of myths about veganism that have made it seem bizarre, cultish, or dangerous.

It is imperative that people recovering from eating disorders who choose to become vegan help to clarify the motivation and practice of veganism and separate the two issues. Veganism is not a malady. It is a vibrant, healthful lifestyle and philosophy based on a reverence for all life, which includes animals, the earth, all humans, and oneself.

Reproduction and Human Health

Should vegans have children?

The choice to have children or not is a very personal decision, one that cannot be based on the vegan ethic alone. There are many issues that vegans must weigh, including the advantages versus the liabilities of bringing new life into the world. It is also important to understand the motivation behind our desire to conceive and raise children and to determine if alternatives with greater benefits than drawbacks exist that would satisfy our needs just as effectively.

In a democratic society, the notion of mandatory reproductive restrictions is anathema. Forced sterilization and birth control were outlawed many years ago in the United States, even for those with impaired judgment or a limited capacity to make reasonable decisions for themselves, such as people with mental illness or mental retardation. Reproductive freedom is perceived as an inalienable right, and this viewpoint is unlikely to change in the foreseeable future. Furthermore, some faiths laud the birth of a child as a gift from the Creator and, in a society that extols religious autonomy, there are few who would debate this prerogative. When sovereignty over one's body is considered fundamental, and when children are viewed as blessings, not burdens, it is impossible to impose limitations on human procreation. Vegans represent a wide range of spiritual and theological viewpoints; thus it would be impossible to achieve consensus among vegans on the rightness or wrongness of having children from a legal or religious perspective.

Because few cultures impose regulations on reproduction, the human population is expanding at a phenomenal rate. According to estimates by the U.S. Census Bureau, the U.S. population increased by approximately 47 million people from 1977 to 1997. At a current annual growth rate of 2.4 million people, the U.S. population will continue to expand by more than 2 million people a year well into the twenty first century. Worldwide, the human population is increasing by an astounding 80 million people a year.

It took all of human history for the population to reach its first billion in 1800. The second billion only took until 1930. Today, more than six billion people crowd the planet. These figures are staggering and should call attention to the labyrinth of consequences linked to the explosion of our species. More people means:

- rising demands for housing, resulting in greater loss of native flora, habitat, and wildlife;

- escalating consumption of nonrenewable natural resources;
- widespread congestion in cities, suburbs, and on roadways;
- increased environmental degradation and pollution;
- elevated energy demands;
- more unhoused people and abandoned children;
- reduced access to basic necessities;
- diminished community; and
- a greater dichotomy between the haves and have-nots.

A number of social scientists concede that the majority of our modern problems–ecological imbalance, environmental destruction, species extinction, rage, violence, hunger, poverty, homelessness–stem from our inability to control the growth of our own population. Granted, this is not the sole cause of our current environmental crises and social dilemmas, but it appears to be at least a contributing factor that vegans must not overlook.

A few organizations have been working for decades to mitigate population growth. Unfortunately, their success has been minimal. Education, easy access to contraceptives, and encouraging adoptions instead of new births are all prudent means to control population that vegans can consider. In a free society, other possibilities are unthinkable.

Each individual's circumstances, rationale, and motivation for having or not having children are unique, so there can be no definitive answer to the question. Nevertheless, vegans (and nonvegans alike) should evaluate the issues and statistics prior to making a choice about parenthood. Having children means creating more people, which can only exacerbate our existing problems. Even if we believe that vegan children will be more aware or better equipped to solve the world's problems, we all must weigh the consequences against any expected benefit from reproduction.

Whether or not vegans become birth parents, there are endless opportunities to nurture youngsters, including adopting, caring for the children of relatives, friends, or neighbors, foster parenting, mentoring, becoming a big brother or big sister, or doing volunteer work. We can also nurture the life around us–plants, animals, and people–thereby encouraging a more hospitable, habitable, informed, and loving world.

What is the official vegan stance on abortion?

No moral dilemma exists that is quite like the issue of abortion. A fetus grows within and is dependent on the pregnant woman carrying it, so the situation is distinctly different from that of animals or humans already born and conspicuously alive. Simple observation readily confirms the obvious with regard to the suffering of people and animals. The question of whether life originates at conception, later in gestation, or at birth is an enigmatic matter that has sparked passionate political, legal, and ecclesiastical debate.

Vegans are all across the board in their view of abortion. Although many vegans feel that abortion is a relevant vegan issue, there is no consensus of opinion. Even vegans who have parallel points of view on most matters often come to very different conclusions on this one. This is because determining when life begins is a complex and subjective affair, one that frequently involves spiritual or religious considerations. Consequently, this issue is just as contentious and no easier to resolve within the bounds of veganism than it is in the general public.

Veganism is not a theology and, accordingly, vegans come from a diverse range of backgrounds and outlooks. Because vegans do not share a uniform position on abortion, there is no "official stance." This matter is best resolved by individual practitioners in the context of their personal perspectives or spiritual beliefs.

Do vegans only refrain from using and consuming nonhuman products, or are human products included as well? For instance, do vegans abstain from organ transplants and blood transfusions?

Organs that are used for transplantation are removed from human donors at the time of or shortly after death. This contribution is based on the wishes of benefactors prior to their demise or the consent of the deceased's family. Anguish is rarely provoked by the donation of an organ. Organs for transplantation typically come from healthy, relatively young individuals who die suddenly and prematurely. The families of organ donors generally take comfort in knowing that their relative's death may provide fresh hope for someone in dire distress. Consequently, there is no philosophical conflict between veganism and human-to-human organ transplantation.

Blood transfusions are no different from organ donations except that the contributors are still living and have willingly supplied their blood. There is no harm or suffering incurred by giving or accepting human blood. To the contrary, donating blood is a generous, life-saving gift.

There is purpose and wisdom associated with vegan practice. Shunning bodily substances from other people simply because they are animal products doesn't make sense. From such a narrow vantage point, vegans would be prohibited from nursing their children, having sexual intercourse, or even kissing. Certainly this is not the intent of vegan living.

In a democratic society, people have free will and can give permission for their body parts or fluids to be used. When there is no coercion or exploitation involved, and an arrangement is devised that is agreeable to all parties, there is no question of incompatibility with veganism. Indeed, voluntarily providing assistance to others in need through the use of our bodies is an act of mercy that epitomizes the heart of vegan practice and is a quintessential example of empathy in action.

When talking about the physical differences between carnivores and humans, some people have mentioned that we have the physical characteristics of both carnivores and herbivores and therefore were meant to eat meat. Even though we have more characteristics of herbivores, it is assumed that since we have a few carnivorous attributes, it follows that meat should be included in our diet. How would you tackle this? I have quoted the following differences:

- We do not have a hinged jaw for ripping apart flesh but one that is able to grind sideways.
- We have a longer digestive system so we are better able to get

nutrients from our foods, as opposed to the shorter tract that carnivores have to enable them to pass meat through their body before it becomes rancid.

- The low levels of acidity in our stomachs are in stark contrast to the high levels in meat-eaters.
- Although we have incisors capable of tearing flesh, I have always thought that these were for cropping the harder vegetables.
- We do not have claws or talons for tearing flesh.
- The enzymes in our saliva that start breaking down food have a low acidity level related to a plant-based diet.

There has been much dissension among scientists regarding the topic of human physiology and diet, and opinions have spanned the continuum from one end to the other. The fact is, human physiology does not fit neatly into any of the three major categories of mammalian diets: carnivorous, herbivorous, or omnivorous. We have a few traits from each of these classifications, which makes it easy for researchers to prove their position merely by pointing out those characteristics that suit their particular opinion.

It is often suggested that specific features of human anatomy or physiology dictate our behavior. However, from the perspective of diet, our physical makeup only prescribes our nutritional requirements, not from which sources specific nutrients must be obtained.

The argument that biology is destiny is typically used to justify a particular eating style. In that light, we must acknowledge that humans are the only species on earth that appears to have no idea what its ideal diet should be. Nutrition science has yet to determine the optimal eating plan for human beings. Our confusion is readily evidenced by the weight-loss, supplement, and diet crazes that sprout up and fade away with predictable regularity. Even among those who follow plant-based diets there is disagreement about whether a low-fat, raw foods, high-protein, macrobiotic, or other eating style is best. We are also the only species that has self-inflicted diet-related diseases, that causes extensive environmental destruction through basic food production, and that creates pathogenic infestations that widely infect our food supply.

This type of reasoning also blatantly ignores a critical element of human evolution–the aspect of choice. The arguments that "humans are meant to eat meat" and "humans have always eaten meat" are certainly no rationale to continue the practice. If we were to accept this type of twisted logic, we would also have to say that humans have always murdered, raped, enslaved, and committed other heinous acts that our culture today finds reprehensible. Unlike most other animals, humans can choose which foods to eat.

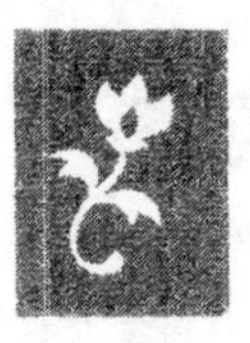

Humans are the only species on earth that appears to have no idea what its ideal diet should be.

Our ability to digest a wide variety of foods undoubtedly contributed to our species' survival throughout history. Today, however, our dietary choices have more to do with tradition, culture, economics, politics, and availability than with some predetermined fate. It is time for our species to behave responsibly and select those foods that best sustain the earth, the animals, and ourselves. Only then can we truly say that humans have evolved in body, spirit, and wisdom.

Dairy and Eggs

What's wrong with organic milk and dairy products? I assume that the farmers don't give their cows drugs and hormones, which makes the milk more healthful. But aren't the animals on organic dairy farms also treated much better?

Veganism is a matter of conscience, not health. Because the motivation for vegans to avoid dairy products is based on principle, it becomes irrelevant how healthful or unhealthful dairy foods may be. Even if dairy cows were treated like royalty, they will still be killed after living only a fraction of their normal life span. When a farmer says his or her animals are organically raised, it does not necessarily mean that the animals are treated more humanely or given more space for movement and housing.

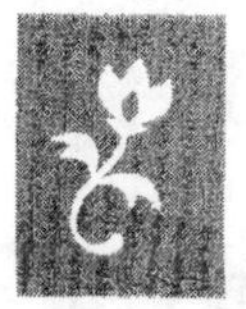

Veganism is a matter of conscience, not health.

On organic dairy farms, as on factory-style dairies, cows must be kept continually pregnant. The cycle begins when a heifer's body is barely mature enough to withstand the burden of bearing a calf. Dairy cows are mammals and, like all mammals, they naturally produce milk for a period of time after giving birth to feed their young. Gestation for cows lasts for nine months and on the average they lactate for ten months. To increase profits and maximize milk production, cows are forced to bear a calf each year, are milked for seven months of their pregnancy, and are reimpregnated via artificial insemination shortly after giving birth. This keeps their milk production strong so they can generate the abnormal yields required to "earn their keep." Moreover, the male calves from organic farms are doomed to the same fate as those from factory-style dairy farms: they will be killed at birth, sold for veal, or raised for beef.

Whether a dairy cow is organically raised or not, she will still be regularly confined, artificially inseminated, endure endless pregnancies and births, forced to produce massive quantities of milk that will be mechanically retrieved, never nurse or enjoy her offspring, subjected to the horrors of transport, and face a cruel and untimely death. Vegans do not use dairy products because they do not consider them a natural food for human beings and because viewing animals as commodities—regardless of whether they live on organic or factory-style farms—inevitably causes needless suffering.

What is the vegan position on free-range eggs?

Free-range is not a legal industry term; therefore it is essentially meaningless. Farmers use the term to imply that they practice a more humane standard of production, but in reality there is no regulation regarding how the word is interpreted. Although most consumers imagine free-range hens have access to the outdoors with plenty of sunlight, vegetation, and normal social interaction, to most egg producers, the "range" is simply a bigger cage than those in which battery-caged hens are kept. (A battery cage is the 16-inch-wide wire enclosure used in all intensive egg-laying facilities. Although a hen's wingspan is 30 to 32 inches, four to six hens are typically crowded into each cage, making it impossible for the birds to stretch their wings or walk.)

Free-range egg farming is, above all else, a business. Consequently, profit surpasses concern for the animals' comfort, welfare, or behavioral needs. In addition, it is common for free-range layers (egg-producing hens) to be debeaked just like battery-caged layers. Debeaking involves crudely amputating portions of the hens' beaks, cutting through bone, cartilage and delicate soft tissue. This ghastly procedure–performed so that distraught hens in cramped quarters won't injure each other and thereby obliterate the farmer's financial investment–is usually administered without the use of anesthesia, even though it is acknowledged that it is exceedingly painful.

But even if free-range hens were treated with kindness and given all the space they could use, they will still be killed for meat when their egg production wanes, usually after one or two years, even though in a natural environment a hen could live about fifteen years. And, like all other animals raised for food, they will be subjected to the horrors and abuses of transportation, handling, and slaughter.

When we treat sentient beings as commodities we invariably invite abuse.

An inherent problem with *all* egg production, whether free-range or battery-caged, is the disposal of unwanted male chicks at the hatchery. Because male chicks don't lay eggs and do not grow fast enough to be raised profitably for meat, they are deemed a financial liability, except for the few used as rooster studs. On average, one rooster is used to service ten hens. Hence, nine out of ten male chicks are considered virtually useless and will be killed by the cheapest means available, including suffocation and being ground up alive.

No matter what words or systems are used to candy-coat animal production, when we treat sentient beings as commodities, we invariably invite abuse. From a vegan perspective, the use of animals for human profit or gain, regardless of how they are raised or treated, is incompatible with vegan principles and the practice of compassionate living.

If I had a house in the mountains where I owned a cow and a chicken that had been abandoned, would it be okay to drink the cow's milk and eat the chicken's eggs?

Vegans oppose the consumption of cow's milk and bird's eggs for many reasons, not only because the majority of cows and chickens are kept on factory farms. Underlying your scenario is the assumption that vegans crave cow's milk and bird's eggs and would consume them if only the animals who produce them were kept in more "humane" conditions. Vegans do not eat these items because they do not consider them to be natural foods for humans.

Vegans also do not view cows and birds as machines and do not believe their milk or eggs should be used as commodities. The aberrant reproductive capacities of cows and chickens have been contrived through genetic engineering, drugs, hormones, rich feed, artificial insemination, and environmental manipulation. In a natural setting, a cow would lactate only to nourish her calf until it was weaned, and chickens would produce eggs at a drastically reduced rate. For example, in 1933, hens laid an average of 70 eggs a year. Today, a four-pound factory-farmed hen averages 275 eggs per year.

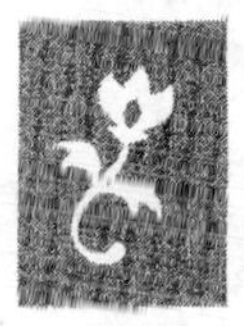

Animal commodities merely serve the purpose of satiating human appetites at the expense of animal welfare and freedom.

Cow's milk and chicken's eggs do not provide people with any nutrients that aren't available in plant foods. Therefore, the only pretext for using them is habit. There are numerous plant foods and items made from them that easily take the place of dairy products and eggs for all purposes. No one need sacrifice familiar flavors, textures, or nutrition to be vegan.

Rationalizing the use of dairy products and eggs because the animals are kept in our own backyard merely endorses the continued enslavement of animals for human desire. It also encourages an ongoing but superfluous reliance on animal-based foods, stimulates a growing demand for these items, and opens the door to avarice, all of which contributed to the instigation of our deplorable factory farm situation in the first place.

Insects and Sea Life

Does being vegan include not harming insects? I could give up honey and stop wearing silk, but what would be the point unless I also stop swatting mosquitos, flea-dipping my cats, and removing wasp nests from my living quarters? Do most vegans do this?

Insects are included under the vegan umbrella of life, and deliberately harming or killing insects is contrary to vegan philosophy. Infrequently, it is necessary to eradicate insects to preserve our health or safety or that of those we love. It is a common response to swat at mosquitos or other biting or stinging insects, although we can retrain ourselves to react differently. In the case of a swarm, attack, or bodily invasion, such as with fleas, humane solutions are often insufficient and more forceful methods must be employed.

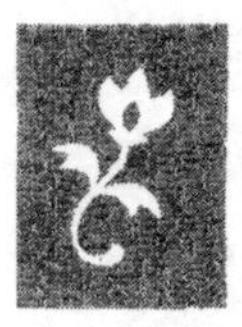

It is illogical to justify the harming of one group of individuals simply because we cannot avoid harming another group.

There is a significant difference between halting storming insects and using honey or silk. When we or our loved ones are under siege and our lives or health are at stake, we must use whatever resources are available to stop it. Honey and silk, on the other hand, are unnecessary luxuries for which numerous vegan alternatives exist.

It is illogical to justify the harming of one group of individuals simply because we cannot avoid harming another group. With this kind of rationalization, we could simiiarly say that since we cannot avoid stepping on ants in the grass, we may as well eat beef. There is no correlation between one and the other. As vegans, we do what we can to live a harm-free existence. But simply because we cannot do so perfectly does not warrant the dissolution of vegan practice.

Why don't vegans consume honey?

There is a prevalent misconception that honeybees are native to the Americas. Most research, however, indicates that honeybees originated in Africa and were introduced to the United States by European colonists.

Honey is made from sucrose-rich flower nectar that is collected by honeybees and then regurgitated back and forth among them until it is partially digested. After the final regurgitation, the bees fan the substance with their wings until it is cool and thick. This is the substance that we call honey, a rich source of carbohydrates that is the principal food source of the hive.

The bees eat some of the honey immediately after it is produced; the remainder is stored in special cells for future use. A natural nest has roughly a hundred thousand cells that comprise half a dozen combs made of beeswax. It takes about fifteen pounds of honey for worker bees to synthesize the wax that goes into such a structure. Some of the cells will be used to store honey and pollen while others, called brood cells, will hold the unborn workers, drones, and infant queens. Honey and pollen are the principal food sources of the developing larvae. Honey is not only vital for sustaining the life cycle of the hive, it provides essential food energy throughout the year, especially during the winter months when nectar and pollen are unavailable.

Winter is a critical time for honeybees. Unlike many other insects, honeybees do not become dormant in cold weather. Instead, they create a warm microclimate inside the hive and live on the stored honey. To maintain a subsistence temperature of about 50 degrees in the outermost layer of the hive and a much higher temperature at the core, worker bees beat their wings to produce heat. During this time the colony must consume about two pounds of honey per week from the more than forty pounds of stored honey to maintain the hive's temperature and ensure the colony's survival during the cold months.

During the collection of flower nectar the bees also pollinate plants. This is a vital part of the natural process of life. Even though humans inadvertently benefit, the bees do not pollinate plants to serve human needs; it is simply an ancillary aspect of their nectar collecting. The majority of our native wild pollinators have been decimated through loss of habitat, environmental degradation, and disease. As a result, today's agriculture relies heavily on wild and kept colonies of honeybees for pollination. Nonetheless, the issues of human consumption of bee products (such as honey, beeswax, pollen, propolis, and royal jelly) and plant pollination are mutually exclusive. Bees would pollinate crops regardless of human economic motives or tastes. Even though we presently depend on kept colonies of honeybees as pollinators, this in no way necessitates our ravaging their hives. There is absolutely no reason to take honey from bees other than to exploit their efforts for our financial gain.

The vegan position on honey is definitive. Honey was prohibited for use by vegans according to the 1944 manifesto of the British Vegan Society (veganism's founding organization), a position consistent with the requirement for full membership in the American Vegan Society since its inception in 1960.

What is wrong with eating oysters and mussels?

Mussels and oysters are part of the enormously successful phylum of mollusks, translated from the Latin name *Mollusca*. Mollusks, sometimes called the "soft ones," constitute one of the most advanced groups of animals in the invertebrate world. In general terms, mollusks are soft-bodied, unsegmented, shell-bearing invertebrates (animals without backbones). Living mollusks comprise seven classes that are as different from each other as a mammal is from a bird.

Virtually all animals that constitute more than one cell have some sort of nervous system or nerve net. Although most mollusks do not have a well-developed brain, they do have highly developed ganglia, which are knots or collections of nerve cells. Some mollusks, such as octopuses, do have very complex brains and possess intelligence levels that have proved greater than those of many vertebrates. In addition, they have long- and short-term memories, as do vertebrates. Most mollusks are slow-moving or sedentary; however, a few, such as the squids, are among the swiftest travelers. Various species of mollusks can burrow in mud, wood, or stone; a number can swim; others can crawl or jump. Their eating habits also vary widely. Some are carnivorous, some are vegetarians, and some are scavengers.

All mollusks have one or more faculties for protection or defense, such as shelly armor, acute senses of smell and touch, keen sight, strong muscles, tunneling skills, or the capability to discharge a caustic inky fluid. These distinctive attributes are evidence of the mollusks' ability to experience and respond to pain or fear and escape or protect themselves from danger.

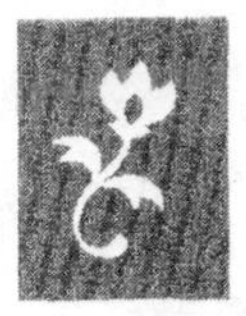

For vegans, the issue isn't finding a reason not to kill but learning what it means to honor life.

Mollusks and all sea animals are diverse and unique creatures whose right to live freely, unencumbered by human interference, is acknowledged and respected by the vegan ethic. There is every scientific reason to believe these animals value their lives, as do all sentient beings, feel pain, demonstrate fear, and want to live. Philosophic veganism espouses a reverence for the totality of life. This conviction includes sea animals no less than any others.

Some of my vegetarian friends have given up their vegetarian diet to go back to eating fish. What is unethical about eating fish?

Fish are not plants. They are sentient living beings that have a heart, brain, and central nervous system, and, as such, they feel pain, suffer, and struggle to stay alive. There are life forms that spend most of their time in the air, some that dwell in trees, others that roam the earth, and still others that inhabit our waterways. Whether an individual has fur, feathers, skin, or scales; lungs or gills; or legs, wings, or fins, her or his life is as dear and meaningful as any other. When fish are caught, their pain is quite apparent to anyone who is even mildly observant. They scream in ways we cannot hear but can easily see. They violently gasp for breath as they drown in our sea of oxygen. They skirt harm whenever possible. And they visibly value their lives no less than we value ours.

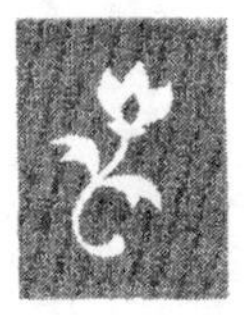

Vegans accept on faith that all living beings treasure their lives.

For vegans, the issue isn't finding a reason not to kill but learning what it means to honor life. When it comes to such grievous matters, we cannot risk being even slightly mistaken because the outcome is so utterly devastating and irrevocable. Vegans accept on faith that all living beings, including fish, treasure their lives. There is no sound reason to believe otherwise, and to behave as if this weren't true would be, for vegans, untenable.

Leather and Animal Fibers

As a vegetarian (one who eats dairy), is it okay to wear leather? The first thing people say when I tell them I am a vegetarian is: If you wear leather, it is the same thing as eating animals. What is the correct response to this, if there is one?

If your decision to be a vegetarian includes the ethical principle of compassion, you owe it to yourself and your conscience to fully understand the interconnectedness of animal commodities. The blunt truth is that the meat, leather, and dairy industries are tangibly and economically intertwined.

The animal-based materials that are prevalent in a culture are determined by the principal meat industries. For instance, in Australia, where kangaroo meat is utilized, particularly in the pet food industry, kangaroo leather is used fairly extensively for handbags, accessories, and tourist items such as stuffed toy kangaroos and koalas, as well as for kangaroo-skin rugs. In other parts of the world where sheep meat is favored, sheepskin, shearling, and wool are rampant. In North America, cattle are the predominant food animals. Not surprisingly, leather, the skin of these animals, is widely used.

It is economically foolish for the slaughter industries to toss away profitable animal parts, so essentially every appendage, muscle, and organ is baked, boiled, ground, or otherwise processed into a salable product. The leather industry is virtually reliant on the beef industry. The beef industry rakes in even greater profits because of its ties with the leather industry.

Dairy cows survive only a fraction of their normal lifespan. In a natural environment cattle can live up to twenty-five years. On modern dairy farms, however, cows are considered spent–drained, worn out, and useless–between four and six years of age. After enduring incredible physical abuse and stress, these relatively young cows are unable to continue to produce sufficient milk or offspring to remain lucrative for the farmers. Considered an economic liability, they are shipped off to slaughter. About one-fifth of all hamburger meat in the United States is made from the flesh of spent dairy cows. Their hides are used in the production of leather, comprising the largest percentage of the so-called by-products of dairying and meat processing.

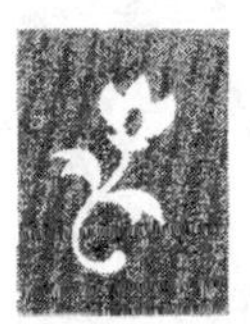

The leather industry is virtually reliant on the meat and dairy industries for a continual supply of animal parts for its raw materials.

Another horrifying aspect of these industries is the use of male calves. Dairy cows are impregnated at a very young age–sometimes even before their bodies are mature enough to endure the strain of pregnancy–in order to make the animals as profitable as possible as soon as possible. They are then artificially inseminated shortly after giving birth, a grueling cycle that continues throughout their unnaturally shortened lives.

Half the calves born will be male, which are of no use to the dairy farmer. They are, however, considered valuable to the beef, veal, and leather industries. The majority of male calves are auctioned to beef producers. Others will be sold to the vicious veal industry, where some will be killed immediately to be used to make cheaper-grade veal products. Others will be sent to veal farms to live out brief, tortured existences, deprived of their mother's milk and comfort and denied virtually all sensory stimulation. Cruel isolation and deprivation methods are employed because these techniques keep the calves' flesh tender and white, thereby commanding a higher price. When the calves are only twelve to sixteen weeks old, they will be slaughtered for the gourmet veal market.

The soft, unblemished hides of these little calves are considered quite valuable. They are used in making expensive calfskin shoe uppers, gloves, wallets, and other costly accessories. Some dairy cows are sent to slaughter while they are pregnant. It is not uncommon for industry workers to abort the baby calves or remove them after the mothers are slaughtered. The delicate, unmarred skin of unborn and newly born calves is considered the finest and most luxurious.

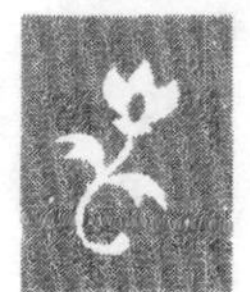

From an ethical perspective, leather, dairy products, and meat are indistinguishable.

Does purchasing leather goods contribute, even in some small measure, to the support and perpetuation of the meat industry? Unquestionably, yes. The use of leather also helps sustain the dairy industry, which is responsible for creating and maintaining the veal industry. The use of dairy products, in turn, helps subsidize the meat and leather industries. It is a brutal cycle of cruelty and death among industries that are financially interdependent and reliant on each other for a continual supply of animal parts for their raw materials.

In many ways, using leather is comparable to eating meat. Leather is a by-product of the meat industry. Therefore, the purchase of leather goods contributes directly to the continued slaughter of billions of animals used for meat each year.

People who choose to be vegetarians because they do not want to participate in the senseless killing of animals for food must seriously evaluate the impact of all their lifestyle choices if they want to maintain a consistent philosophy. From an ethical perspective, leather, dairy products, and meat are indistinguishable.

Is silk vegan?

Silk is not vegan. It is a viscous protein substance secreted from the glands of silkworms that hardens into silk on contact with air. This soft, lustrous fiber is obtained from the cocoon of the silkworm. To retain a single unbroken filament, the silkworm is killed before it can emerge from the cocoon and break the thread. Slaughtering silkworms for their silk is done by boiling, baking, or steaming the live worm directly in its cocoon. When the worm is in this chrysalis stage it is not dead; it is transforming. Therefore, we must believe on faith that its sentience remains intact. To assume otherwise would be unconscionable.

Selective breeding over many generations has expunged the moth's ability to fly. Certain chrysalises are kept aside to allow the moths to emerge and mate. After the female lays her eggs, she is crushed and inspected for diseases. If she appears diseased, her eggs are immediately destroyed. After mating, the males are dumped into a basket and discarded as refuse. According to research conducted by Beauty Without Cruelty (India), approximately fifteen hundred chrysalises are killed to produce one hundred grams of pure silk.

Depending on the weave, style, design, or place where it is woven, silk may be called different names in the marketplace. Some common names for certain types of woven silk are pure chiffon, pure georgette, organza, pure crepe, pure satin, and raw silk. To confuse matters further, chiffon, georgette, crepe, and satin may also be made of synthetic fibers. When buying clothing, ties, handkerchiefs, handbags, hats, ribbons, curtains, upholstered furniture, embroidered items, and typewriter and printer ribbons, check the label for fabric content.

Why don't vegans wear wool?

On the surface it appears that wool is a benign product because, at least theoretically, it can be obtained without harming the sheep. However, upon closer inspection we find that the wool industry is actually very similar to the egg and dairy industries. Although animals such as laying hens, dairy cows, and wool-bearing sheep are not immediately killed to procure their salable products, they suffer tremendously for years prior to their slaughter.

Most people believe that sheep are overburdened with too much wool and therefore need to be shorn. Although today's wool-bearing sheep have thick, heavy coats, it is the result of selective breeding over hundreds of years. These animals are descended from wild mountain sheep, still found in some remote regions of the world, which shed their fine woolly hair naturally. Wool provides sheep with warmth and protection from inclement weather and sunburn. Consequently, modern wool-bearers are extremely vulnerable to the elements when they are denuded.

From the earliest times there was complicity in the use of wool. Merinos, which were originally from Spain, are the most efficient wool producers. Mutton breeds, which primarily originated in England, are used predominately for meat. Cross-breeds are raised for the dual purpose of meat and wool. Nevertheless, Merinos also yield mutton and mutton breeds also yield wool. No sheep escapes either function; it is just a matter of emphasis. Essentially all wool is a slaughterhouse product.

The purchase of wool supports the annual slaughter of millions of lambs and sheep for meat. Essentially all wool is a slaughterhouse product.

Wool is classed as either "shorn wool," which is shorn from sheep annually, or "pulled wool," which is taken from sheep at the time of slaughter. Horrors abound on sheep farms, including painful mutilating surgical procedures that are performed without anesthesia. A large percentage of the world's wool is produced from Merinos exported from Australia. These sheep are crammed onto ships by the tens of thousands, crowded into filthy pens, and packed so tightly they can barely move. As a result, thousands of sheep die each year from suffocation, trampling, or starvation while in transport.

Sheep shearers are paid at a piece rate, meaning that speed, not precision, guides the process. Consequently, most sheep are roughly handled, lacerated, and injured during shearing.

The production of wool, as with all industries that consider animals mere commodities, is rife with suffering and abuse. In addition, the purchase of wool supports the slaughter of millions of lambs and sheep each year. It is for these reasons that vegans do not use wool or any other fibers obtained from animals.

Companion and Captive Animals

Please address the philosophical debate about having companion animals in the home. I struggle with the idea that I have adopted cats and now confine them to my home. Although I love the cats, they are not in my home by choice.

Most domestic animals, such as dogs and cats, are the result of many years of meticulous inbreeding manipulated by humans for specific purposes. Special physical characteristics and personality traits have made certain breeds particularly amenable to serving human desires. For example, some animals are suited to guard and defend, others are valued for their hunting skills, some win awards in contests and shows, others are esteemed for their warmth and gentleness, and still others are prized as status symbols. These animals are not the same stock as their wild ancestors and, as a result, have become virtually dependent on us for their care and existence. There is essentially no natural habitat to which these animals can return.

Humans have bred and overbred certain varieties of domestic animals so that many of their once alluring features have become precursors to crippling afflictions and deadly disorders. Typically, those that are not up to snuff at birth are discarded, abandoned, or killed by crude and brutal methods. The excuse is that these animals are too expensive to house and feed in relation to the meager selling price the breeders might collect.

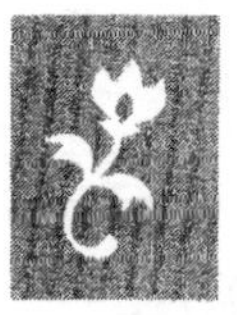

There is essentially no natural habitat
to which domestic companion animals can return.

Shelters are generally packed with both rejected purebreds and unwanted mixed breeds. Making matters worse are irresponsible guardians who deliberately breed their domestic animals, permit wanton intercourse, or refuse to have them spayed or neutered. Our cities, parks, and wooded and rural areas are teeming with unwanted animals who are desperate for food and shelter, constantly exposed to the harsh elements, and easy targets for predation, torture, poisoning, highway death, and seizure.

The majority of shelters euthanize healthy animals that have not been adopted within a week or two. No-kill shelters–those that house animals indefinitely—have limited space, are expensive to operate, and usually have lengthy waiting lists of animals in need of assistance and sanctuary.

The decision to take in a homeless animal is a deeply personal one, and there are many factors to weigh. Adopting an animal is not unlike adopting a child—it is a huge responsibility. Some domestic animals can live for twenty years or longer, so adopters must be prepared for a long-term commitment. Occasionally animals require special food or care, medical attention, or medication. Treatment of certain conditions may be costly, or food requirements could conflict with a person's vegan values. Lifestyle, habits, and work and travel schedules all become important considerations when deciding to adopt an animal companion.

It is irresponsible for people to disregard the cries of homeless or abandoned animals. A compassionate perspective calls for aiding them in whatever way we can. For some vegans this means actively striving to close breeding mills and the pet stores that support them. For others it means contributing to no-kill shelters through donations of money or food, or volunteering to walk dogs, clean cages, and spend time playing with and giving attention to the animals. Many grassroots animal activist groups have, or would be interested in starting, a local spay and neuter program, which could be coordinated with city government or animal control agencies. And, of course, there is always the option of adopting a companion animal in need.

Some vegans feel that taking an animal into their home is comparable to imprisonment. The blunt truth is that the animals have nowhere else to go. Nevertheless, most people find that sharing their lives with animals is a reciprocally gratifying and beneficial arrangement, one that encourages a deeper appreciation for other life forms and inspires a unique bond of friendship and trust that transcends all barriers of language and form.

What is the vegan perspective on feeding companion animals meat?

There is no "official" vegan position regarding what to feed companion animals and the vegan community is conflicted over this issue. Dogs and cats are the primary topic of contention, since the majority of other animal companions are, by nature, herbivorous.

Dogs are able to eat a wide variety of foods and, with proper supplementation, many can do well on a predominately plant-based diet. Cats, however, require meat to thrive.

There are no long-term studies or solid scientific data to support putting cats on vegan diets. Any presumed benefits are simply conjecture promulgated primarily by the manufacturers of these products and well-meaning activists. However, scientific and anecdotal information regarding the hazards abound. We do not have hard evidence yet to ascertain whether synthetic essential nutrients are metabolized effectively by felines. It is quite possible that a number of cats fed a vegan diet could appear to be healthy for several years and then suddenly experience devastating health- or life-threatening consequences.

Vegans and vegetarians often like to underscore the anatomical differences between carnivores and herbivores to support their belief that humans are not designed to eat meat. They are also repulsed and furious that some "food animals," such as cows, which are total vegetarians, are commonly fed ground-up animal products or even their own species. If we believe it is wrong for natural vegetarians to be force-fed meat, the inverse should be equally morally objectionable. Cows are designed to eat plant matter; cats are designed to eat flesh.

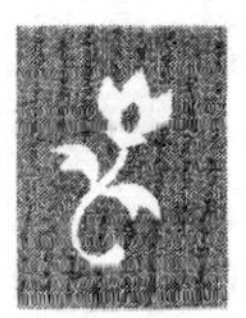

There are no perfect feeding solutions when our companion animals are carnivores.

Humans have a choice about their ethics and the foods that they eat; our companion animals do not. They are compelled to eat what we provide for them, even though they inherently know what their bodies require. Place a hungry cat in a room with an apple and a mouse, and the cat will instinctively go after the mouse and ignore the apple. Sometimes vegans deprive their cats of alternative foods for long periods just so the animal will eat a plate of oats and lentils—hardly the normal diet for a feline with dagger-like canines, retractable claws, no crushing molars, no sideways-grinding jaw, a short gut, and powerful stomach acids.

There are no perfect feeding solutions when our companion animals are carnivores. Commercial pet foods are the dregs of the slaughterhouse industries and are rife with contaminants. Although organic meat-based cat food is a step up the ladder as far as purity, it still contains discarded animal parts often deemed inedible by humans, and there is no way to guarantee that the animals were not diseased or given drugs prior to their death. No matter how it is analyzed, from an ethical perspective the ingredients in all animal-based pet foods are equally problematic, whether homemade from human-grade organic meats or scooped from a can or bag.

Vegans are entitled to practice and abide by their beliefs and even influence other people to do so, but is it fitting to impose our ethics on another species, especially one that would not oblige us if other options were provided? If some vegans cannot respect a cat's physiology and biological requirements, perhaps they should not adopt felines. Instead, those vegans who are concerned about the welfare of cats but are unwilling to give them the meat-based diet they are designed to consume could work toward eliminating the domestic cat market through implementing extensive spay and neuter programs and breeding bans.

From a moral vantage point, it is critical to analyze all angles of this problem and not settle on an easy resolution simply because on the surface it appears to comply with vegan convictions. We must be realistic about what is truly in the best interests of the animals that are in our custody right now, even if the present solutions are limited and less than ideal.

What is the vegan view on seeing-eye dogs?

There is no definitive vegan position on seeing-eye dogs. Some people may consider these dogs to be in servitude to human beings and, from a certain angle, they are, but certainly no more so than the most beloved companion animal or faithful friend. People who are vision impaired develop an incredible bond with their dogs that is unlike any other interspecies relationship. They literally place their lives in their dog's paws every day, and both are equally reliant on and devoted to each other.

The dogs that are selected to assist vision-impaired people are highly intelligent, easily trained breeds and mixed breeds with affectionate personalities that reflect loyalty, faithfulness, and dependability. They are not abused during their training and are extremely dedicated to their human companions. In return, they are given love and the best care possible. In general, these dogs are highly respected by their trainers, their charges, and the public at large.

Seeing-eye dogs and their vision-impaired humans have a symbiotic alliance based on trust, cooperation, and commitment. From outward observation, it seems to be a mutually rewarding partnership. Still, veganism argues that these animals would not willingly submit to being in human service if given a choice, regardless of how well they are treated.

Utilizing animals to fulfill human needs is in conflict with basic vegan tenets. Despite the benefit to certain groups of people, from a vegan perspective the use of seeing-eye dogs would appear to be insupportable. Nevertheless, because seeing-eye dogs present a unique solution to a challenging problem for which no alternatives presently exist, a conclusive vegan opinion may be impossible. All matters considered, it is reasonable and logical that seeing-eye dogs should simply come under the vegan category of what is neither "practical nor possible" for some vision-impaired people to do without.

Are there enough animals and fish that die of natural causes to feed carnivorous zoo and circus animals so we don't have to slaughter other animals to feed them?

Nature provides intrinsic controls that maintain the delicate balance of life. When an animal dies in a natural setting of natural causes, it is usually because of predation, infirmity, overburdened carrying capacity (the number of creatures that can be sustained by a habitat), or old age. Predators typically go after the most vulnerable individuals, targeting those who are very young, weak, or incapable of keeping up with the herd. This is called "survival of the fittest," which fosters the evolution of stronger species. In general, when animals die in the wild, they are either killed and consumed as prey, or they expire in remote areas where it would be unfeasible to locate and retrieve them. Many others also die at the hands of human poachers, who view the animals only in terms of dollars, or by indirect human interference, such as habitat destruction and pollution.

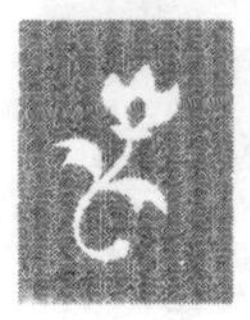

When we remove species from their natural environment, overbreed them, and keep them captive, we distort their lives and imbalance the natural world.

Predator-prey relationships are part of nature. Carnivores are physically designed to hunt, kill, and devour their quarry quickly and painlessly. In their natural habitat, wild animals know exactly what they should eat or on whose menu they might be found. Animals in captivity are denied even these most basic rights and freedoms. When captive carnivores are kept sated by their captors, the animals they might normally hunt and devour become more like playthings, as when a cat stalks and torments a mouse but does not eat it. Situations like this are little more than stunted opportunities for carnivores to minimally exercise their natural abilities while remaining functionally immature and dependent on their human caretakers.

When we remove species from their natural environment, overbreed them, and keep them captive, we distort their lives and imbalance the natural world. There is no restitution that can restore equilibrium to the earth or provide justice for the animals. Our only recourse is to ban animal imports and captive breeding programs, and to disallow further obliteration of habitat and natural resources.

Theory, Polemics, and Politics

I have been a vegetarian for a couple of months now and I am working on becoming vegan. There is no doubt in my heart that the life of an animal is as rich and valuable as that of a human. It certainly feels more natural to pick an apple from a tree than to chop the head off a chicken. Still, many omnivores ask me, "How can you think it's not right to kill an animal but it's okay to kill a plant? What if plants feel pain?" I know this is far-fetched, but these people seem to think this is a justification for eating meat and other animal products. Is there anything I can say to them?

All living creatures consume other living things in order to survive. This is a basic fact of life. Unlike many other animals, however, human beings have a choice about what they eat. For vegans, this choice hinges on the issue of sentience, which is easily ascertained by using plain observation and common sense.

There is no scientific reason to believe that plants bring a consciousness or psychological presence to the world. Plants do not have a brain or central nervous system. Therefore, they lack the fundamental mechanisms to experience pleasure, pain, and suffering. Fear and pain would serve no purpose in plants because they are unable to escape any threat. Consequently, there is no logical basis to support the theory that plants feel pain. The dubious possibility that they might, however, is no justification for killing obviously sentient beings.

Any rational person understands the striking difference between slitting the throat of a sentient animal and plucking a fruit or vegetable. Conscionable people are repulsed by animal slaughter; no one is revolted by gleaning crops. Even if there were grounds for acknowledging a sensate component of plants, vegans consume far fewer resources, including plants, than either people on a meat-based diet or vegetarians who eat eggs and dairy products.

Although vegans could theoretically consume just the fruit of plants instead of whole plants, minute life in the soil, air, and water would still be destroyed. In fact, merely by participating in most activities of modern life we inadvertently harm tiny life forms.

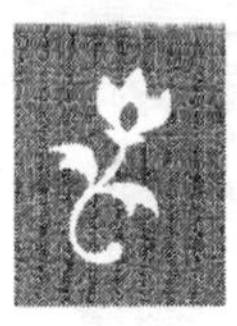

Any rational person understands the striking difference between slitting the throat of a sentient animal and plucking a fruit or vegetable.

This does not mean, however, that vegans should wantonly destroy plant life. The intention to damage or kill violates basic vegan principles. Plants are an essential component of staying alive and remaining healthy. Knowing this, vegans are obliged to grow and use food responsibly; restore and replenish the earth through composting, recycling, and other environmentally caring ways; buy sustainably produced commodities; and take only what is needed.

What would be the official vegan stance on consuming meat from an animal that died of natural causes, such as old age or a natural predator? I was asked this question and found it difficult to answer, save the rather uneducated, "Ick! But it's meat!"

Vegans and vegetarians are commonly baited by nonvegetarians with "what if" scenarios that typically have no relevance to or bearing on most people's real-life situations. Certainly there are unusual circumstances that could challenge a vegan's ability to fully employ her or his beliefs, but these tend to be infrequent exceptions rather than the rule.

All animals eventually die; this is a reality of life. Animals who die in the wild, without human interference, are part of the natural life and death process. Natural selection ensures that the hardiest and healthiest animals outlive the weaker and sicker ones, thereby evolving and strengthening the species. In response to your acquaintance's particular "what if" story, the flesh of an animal that dies of old age would be tough and unpalatable, and the carcass of an animal killed by a natural predator would be devoured or picked apart long before people arrived on the scene. Even if humans found the meat of a very old animal to be appetizing or discovered an intact animal killed by natural predators, they would have to be sitting in wait for the animal's demise to procure the flesh before rigor mortis set in, or it began to putrefy.

This imagined account is based on the erroneous assumption that vegans and vegetarians crave animal flesh, and that they avoid it only because they object to how animals that are raised for food are slaughtered. This suggests that if animals were killed in a more natural or humane fashion, vegans would not only condone eating meat but would desire it. The premise that vegans want or would sanction meat is mistaken. Therefore, the question is intrinsically flawed.

The meat and dairy industries are politically powerful these days. They parallel the tobacco industry of the Seventies. What shocked me is an ad I saw on television for a diet that consists entirely of meat, dairy, and eggs. Watching it appalled me. The thought that kept running through my head was that this program was developed by the meat industry. Who else would advocate such lunacy? Could the meat producers be backlashing against the trend of good nutrition with this plan? Sure smells like it.

More and more nutrition specialists and health care practitioners are recommending diets that include higher amounts of fresh vegetables, whole grains, legumes, and fruits. Consequently, it is not surprising to see those industries that would be most economically damaged by a sweeping move away from animal-based foods react by promoting their products even more aggressively.

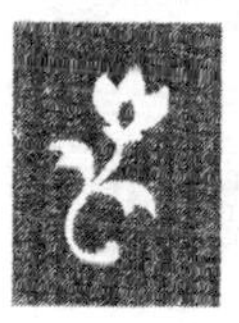

The profusion of vegetarian commodities in the mainstream marketplace is a distinct sign that vegetarianism has arrived.

History has demonstrated that whenever groups of people effect lasting social change, the public passes through three stages: denial and rejection, tolerance, and finally acceptance. Actually, we could interpret this type of audacious advertising in a very positive way. The meat, egg, and dairy industries are no longer able to refute the healthful benefits of a vegan or vegetarian diet, so their only recourse is to champion their products based on whatever premise they can devise. Recent tactics include touting meat as "real food" or "what's for dinner" or painting milk mustaches on celebrities. This also means that the general public is becoming more tolerant of vegetarianism, creating a threatening situation for the brokers of animal-derived foods. It may be a long time before society arrives at stage three, but the profusion of vegetarian commodities in the mainstream marketplace is a distinct sign that vegetarianism has arrived.

As you pointed out, the parallels between the tobacco industry and the meat, egg, and dairy industries are compelling. From personal habit and dependence to public censure, from physician endorsement to open denouncement, from government collusion to levies and lawsuits, meat, eggs, and dairy products are inevitably headed down the same slippery slope as tobacco.

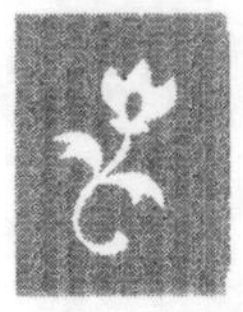

The parallels between the tobacco industry and the meat, egg, and dairy industries are compelling.

However, all these industries are deeply entrenched in our society's economy and way of life. It will take a long while to untangle the practices they have worked so hard to weave into the fabric of our culture.

I agree that these types of ads are shocking and infuriating. But vegans and vegetarians should take heart. View them with a smile and take them with a grain of salt, knowing that because someone felt the need to create such promotions, our movement and influence have been acknowledged.

Global Concerns

I live in a country where the meat comes from Brazil, China, New Zealand, and Australia. Do these countries' meat industries have the same horrible abuse record as the American meat industry?

Regardless of the country, whenever animals are bred and raised for human use and consumption, there is inevitable exploitation. In many countries it is common practice to kill and eat not only cattle, pigs, and birds but also domestic, wild, and exotic animals–such as dogs, horses, goats, dolphins, ostriches, bears, snakes, alligators, and kangaroos, among others–a custom that often appalls even stony North American omnivores. Some cultures utilize barbaric methods of ritual slaughter that involve slitting the throat of a conscious animal and bleeding it to death. Others skin, feather, or boil animals alive. In most parts of the world there are not even the meager health and sanitation policies or inspection procedures that are implemented, albeit minimally, in the United States.

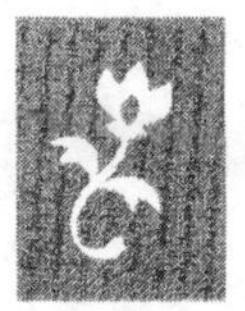

Attaching the word *humane* to any act of extermination turns it into an oxymoron.

No matter how or where an animal is raised for human consumption or which methods are used for slaughter, all animals struggle to stay alive and be free. It is a straightforward and observable fact of life. One country's reprehensible record of abuse does not make it significantly worse than any other country–all are culpable and should be held equally accountable. No standard of killing is notably superior to another because all slaughter ends in suffering and death.

To compare cruelties is a futile intellectual exercise. Brutality and butchering are a matter of intensity and degree, never exoneration. Attaching the word *humane* to any act of extermination merely turns it into an oxymoron. Veganism views all meat as the morbid aftermath of persecution, the country of origin and its history of animal mistreatment notwithstanding.

As a vegan, I am often asked about my lifestyle choice. When I tell people that veganism can be the core solution to so many crucial problems of our day, such as animal suffering, world hunger, water shortages, environmental degradation, loss of rainforest habitat, and species extinction, they want statistics. Can you please help by listing some of the important data?

Many vegans like to flash in-your-face statistics at nonvegans as proof of the superiority of a vegan lifestyle and its potential to save the world. However, most global concerns are complex affairs that involve politics, economics, environmental disputes, cultural misconceptions, racism, ethnocentrism, and more. Although animal commodities contribute to a wide array of problems that affect the welfare of the earth and all living beings, it is difficult to distill the issues down to a few digits. In the end, there are no simple solutions. Veganism may be a sizable piece of the puzzle, but it is only one part of the whole.

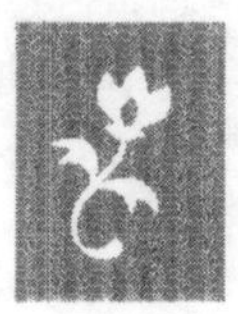

Matters of compassion deal with the essence of our being, not our intellect.

It is incidental whether it's one cow, chicken, pig, or lamb that is slaughtered or one billion. From an environmental perspective, quantities can certainly add up; but from the standpoint of compassion, a single life is always one too many. If people are influenced to change due to impressive numbers, it is just as easy for them to work toward reform and reduction rather than total elimination because an abatement may indeed provide the same functional results. When there is no deep-seated justification for abolishing animal commodities, there is every reason to merely decrease consumption and production rather than eradicate them. This way, people still can have their animals and eat them too.

From the standpoint of compassion, a single life is always one too many.

Unless we focus on issues of pain and suffering and the ethic of compassion, we will forever be subject to the changing tides of research to bolster our position. Matters of compassion deal with the essence of our being, not our intellect. A profound commitment to veganism–the kind that can truly affect the course of the world–will come not from abstract enumerations but from the pulse of our collective hearts.

If every human being became vegan, would the earth be able to produce the food required to feed not only humans but the animals that eat only plants?

Of course. Nature is capable of sustaining all the living creatures of the earth. Primarily, problems have arisen when humans destroy, pollute, or interfere with nature's cycles and processes because we have wrongly assumed that "we can do better" than the natural world pro-

Chapter 2

Relationships

Sowing Seeds of Compassion

Compassion can be described as "empathy in action." Vegans have not cornered the market on compassion—there are many types of compassion and many ways to be compassionate. However, most people construe compassion strictly in terms of human-to-human interaction, and even then often only in light of certain groups. For example, it's common to feel empathic toward children; victims of crime, illness, or tragedy; single mothers; or the elderly. However, some people who express compassion for one group of humans may withhold it from another. For instance, we may be compassionate toward our own ethnic group but not toward someone else's. This does not in any way diminish or devalue the emotion itself nor the positive outcome it might proffer. Nevertheless, the compassion is confined to a very limited segment of the population and, consequently, its ability to ignite inclusive and far-reaching social change is stymied.

Some people do include nonhumans in their circle of compassion, but frequently this involves just a few specific "special interest" animals that may be abused, threatened, or endangered. Other people focus their attention exclusively on domestic companion animals and issues related to their safety, overbreeding, and adoption. Although these pursuits are unquestionably important and have great merit, the scope of the compassion is relatively narrow.

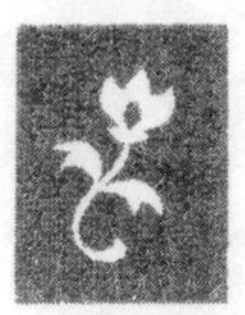

Our cultural conditioning has trained us to respond in predictable patterns of apathy and insensitivity.

There is a degree of irony in selectively applying compassion. It is as if there were truth to the slogan George Orwell's characters in *Animal Farm* came to believe: "All animals are created equal, but some are more equal than others." One example of this paradox is consumers who intentionally purchase dolphin-safe tuna (i.e., tuna fish that were caught and killed without injuring dolphins in the process). Their concern is solely for the dolphins, apparently because they are mammals, like us, with no regard for the dead tuna. Another illustration of incongruous compassion is a bird-watcher who eats poultry. Or an antiabortionist who supports capital punishment. Or an animal rights activist who wears leather shoes.

The vegan ethic stands in stark contrast to convention because it applies compassion indiscriminately. In theory, vegans are concerned about every group or individual who is exploited, human or nonhuman. Although outsiders often view vegan principles as being strict, they are in reality far less stringent than they are consistent.

Implementing a compassionate perspective that embraces all life is at the heart of being vegan. On the surface, this precept sounds reasonable and relatively easy to adopt. In practice, however, it can be quite daunting. Not because there are individuals who are not worthy of respect and justice, but because our cultural conditioning, prejudices, and habits have trained us to respond in predictable patterns of apathy and insensitivity.

Compassion follows only when we come to perceive and value diversity, and when we realize that the life force flowing through us is no different from that which flows through all others.

To become wholly compassionate requires us to open our eyes and hearts, to behold the pain and exploitation our culture obscures, to arouse deadened emotions, and to rise above our egos. This is not an instantaneous transformation, as most of us possess deep-seated intolerances that often reveal themselves only after profound and deliberate examination of our innermost beliefs and feelings. Compassion follows only when we come to perceive and value diversity, and when we realize that the life force flowing through us is no different from that which flows through all others.

Being vegan does not automatically make us more tolerant, more open-minded, more patient, or more loving. However, since vegan principles strongly advocate lifting the social veils of oppression, there is more incentive and opportunity for vegans to grow in their compassion.

Oftentimes compassionate people become so enmeshed in their concern for others that they forget about their own very real and equally valid needs. Because veganism embraces all life, it is essential that we include ourselves in our circle of compassion. Sincerely honoring the vegan ethic dictates that we respect and cherish who we are. Hence, taking time for our physical, emotional, intellectual, and spiritual needs is as crucial as all other vegan actions. Learning to accept or transform our shortcomings and love ourselves by caring for our needs will not only make us more compassionate activists but will make us happier, healthier, and more fulfilled human beings.

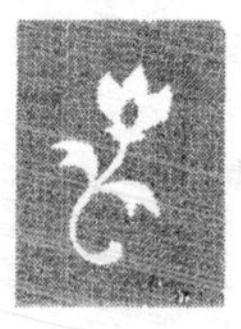

Veganism is not the *totality* of a person's life; it is merely a philosophy that helps shape who we are and how we see the world as we *participate* in life.

Few experiences cause us as much joy, heartache, and confusion as our associations with other people. I have received more questions about vegan practice and the ways in which it affects relationships than any other topic. Our interactions with family, friends, partners, co-workers, neighbors, and acquaintances are worthwhile and valuable. Sadly, sometimes the people closest to us do not understand or appreciate our vegan convictions, and this can be very distressing. Implementing a respectful and understanding approach is difficult when our feelings are hurt, our throat is tight, and our heart feels like a jumbled mass of knots.

Veganism is not the *totality* of a person's life; it is merely a philosophy that helps shape who we are and how we see the world as we *participate* in life. It is hard to maintain a compassionate attitude toward people who are hostile, mean, or belittling to us. But how we respond to them is a large part of being vegan, too. Veganism isn't just about what we avoid–it is about what we think, say, and do. Although this can be a challenge, it is especially important to remember since our thoughts, words, and actions are perhaps more significant and instrumental than all other aspects of being vegan.

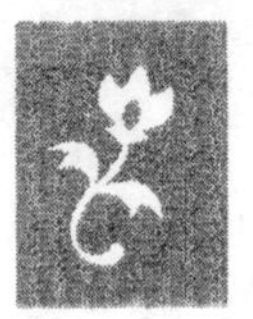

Veganism isn't just about what we avoid—
it is about what we think, say, and do.

Caring for Ourselves

In seeking a compassionate lifestyle and striving to be a conscious vegan, I have often been faced with a problem that I have not yet been able to solve: I have difficulty loving or showing compassion to myself. I am well aware that I can't love others until I love myself, and that not doing so is incongruous with true veganism. What can I do to change this?

Most of us are raised to care about others more than we care about ourselves. Taking time to tend to our own needs is often viewed as a selfish or frivolous indulgence. Breaking away from this indoctrination is difficult, because it generally stems from our earliest training and is a widely accepted point of view.

People who do not care about or respect themselves can easily end up in abusive situations, because they feel they are not worthy of anything better. Some deliberately sabotage relationships, hurt themselves, or humiliate themselves in public to gain attention. People without self-love often strive desperately to be loved by others to compensate for what they cannot give to themselves, or they unconsciously push others away because they do not feel they deserve friends.

Learning to love who we are is an ongoing process. It takes willingness to accept our shortcomings, forgive our blunders, and appreciate our strengths as much as we try to do for others. One of the best places to begin is to change the "tapes" we run through our mind day and night. Instead of berating ourselves when we fumble by thinking "How could you be such a jerk?!" we can tell ourselves, "It was a simple mistake that anyone could have made," or "You did the best you could," or "There are much worse things. This isn't so bad."

Practice dwelling on your positive attributes instead of your drawbacks. Praise yourself silently when you do something well. Make a list of all your strong points and look at it often. Remind yourself of how wonderful you are whenever you feel yourself slipping back into familiar negative patterns.

Occasionally, treat yourself to special excursions: Take yourself out to dinner, read an inspiring book, get a new haircut, take a walk in the park, plant some flowers, meditate under a tree, take dance lessons, study yoga or t'ai chi, learn a musical instrument, teach yourself a new craft, start a journal, or engage in any other activity that you enjoy. Fill your life with fun and observe the beauty that begins to bloom around you. Gently remind yourself to seek out the good in other people and in yourself. Avoid reading about negative local and national news; instead, focus on uplifting material that emphasizes the best in the world.

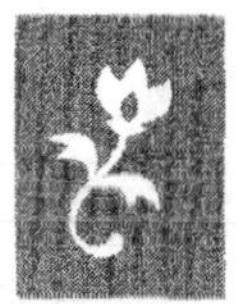

The key to vegan serenity is to strike a comfortable balance between giving to others and giving to oneself.

Commend yourself for having the wisdom, insight, and sensitivity to choose a compassionate lifestyle. Seek out like-minded people who can give you support and encouragement. Join a group that promotes your beliefs and become involved in their activities. Acknowledge that you merit friends and gladness and realize that what you might consider to be flaws may be exactly what someone else sees as endearing. Surround yourself with people who make you smile and laugh. The more humor you bring into your life, the happier you will feel about life in general and yourself in particular. The key to vegan serenity and the prevention of burnout is to strike a comfortable balance between giving to others and giving to oneself.

If, regardless of what you do, you find yourself on an endless downward spiral, know that reaching out for professional help is also an act of self-love and caring. Identifying limitations can be a valuable source of healing, especially if it causes us to seek assistance. Being content with who we are and what we have and understanding our place in the scheme of things can, at times, feel overwhelming. But it is your life, and it is up to you to make it what you want it to be. Do what you need to do in order to feel healthy, whole, and happy. Start with yourself, and all your other acts of compassion will fall appropriately into place.

Do others who are trying to live a vegan lifestyle ever feel deprived? I feel as if I am missing out on so many social events because I can't partake of the food. So much of our society revolves around eating! I feel that I am being selfish to even ask the question—I should be "bigger" than this. Yet I'm aware that I often feel on the outside because I'm not joining in with others. Any suggestions?

Most vegans don't feel deprived as much as they feel estranged when attending nonvegan social functions. Feelings of detachment make sense because there is a very real division between what vegans and nonvegans believe, buy, eat, and do. Food is often used as a way to bond people–whether it's family, friends, or colleagues–because it provides an opportunity to share a pleasant activity and therefore promotes camaraderie. There is a special closeness that develops when people break bread, which is why food is such an important part of celebrations and other social gatherings.

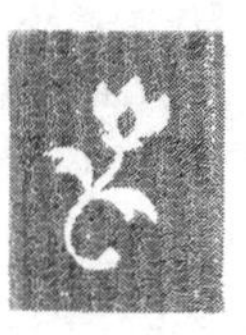

Most vegans don't feel deprived as much as they feel estranged when attending nonvegan social functions.

Feeling left out does not justify compromising one's vegan values. However, it can inspire creative solutions. If you are socializing with people who do not know you are vegan, perhaps it is time to be up front with those you consider to be your friends. If they care about you, they will respect you and honor your choices. If they do not, or if you are afraid to talk to them for fear of rejection, you may want to reevaluate why you have selected them as friends in the first place. True friends will be willing, and often eager, to accommodate a vegan buddy's special needs, sometimes going out of their way to check ingredients, purchase special foods, or prepare a vegan dish. People who cherish you will appreciate this aspect of who you are and will most likely see it as just another quality that makes you the unique and lovable friend that you are.

If you are mingling with people you do not know well or are not close with and you think there will be nothing vegan at the event, chow down beforehand. Food looks much less appealing on a full stomach. You may also want to prepare or buy a special treat for yourself to indulge in once you get home. This way you can think about your goody whenever temptation strikes.

If the people you are mixing with are colleagues from work, you may want to speak privately with the person in charge of food prior to the event and request that a few vegan items be included that everyone could enjoy. You may need to provide suggestions and be willing to purchase or make the food yourself, but this way you would feel confident that you can eat along with everyone else.

Be assertive and look out for your needs. There is no reason to shrink from the crowd or hang your head in silent sadness at the periphery. If you want to be part of the group, reach out and make the first effort. Chances are that your friends have already noticed that you don't eat the food when they are around, and they probably suspect something anyhow. Satisfy their curiosity and your own appetite for food and friendship with the truth. You will all feel sated on a much deeper level.

I like to educate others about the many cruelties inflicted on animals and tell them my reasons for being vegan, but how do I express my views without being so big-headed? I have this idea that my lifestyle somehow makes me and others like me superior to meat-eaters.

Nothing can be taught until the student is ready to learn. Likewise, a teacher who thinks he knows it all rarely does. Vegans are unique in their ability to see our world with clarity and sensitivity for all its inhabitants, and it is easy to feel exalted for being so enlightened. However, there is a vast gulf between seeing and understanding and an even broader chasm between knowledge and wisdom. Wise people are those who realize how little they know.

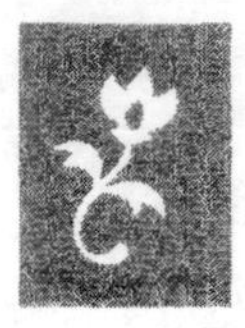

Nothing can be taught until the student is ready to learn.

As humans, our roles of teacher and student are forever reversing and blurring. Most people are more advanced in certain aspects than others, and we all have something to learn from each other. When arrogance about our insights overshadows our sense of humility, how is compassion furthered? No one likes to be told that they are ignorant or uninformed and that someone else holds all the solutions. We each need to grope through life's mysteries in our own way and at our own pace.

It is frustrating to be filled with vital, life-saving information, only to have the people you encounter avoid hearing it. Yet how ready or resistant are you to listen to them in turn? Are you willing to be a captive audience and consider their ideas and follow their suggestions?

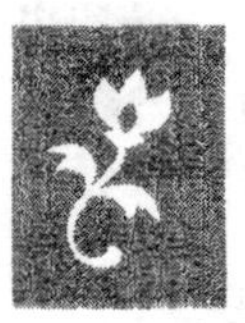

There is a vast gulf between seeing and understanding and an even broader chasm between knowledge and wisdom. Wise people are those who realize how little they know.

We, too, need to remain open, flexible, and attentive if we hope to garner the respect of people whose viewpoints are contrary to our own. We must also remember to reflect the vegan principles of kindness, thoughtfulness, forgiveness, and compassion if our message is to be heeded and our sincerity believed.

I very much admire your work and your views on the reality of veganism, but I wonder how you manage to hedge discouragement.

Doing what you do, I imagine you're surrounded constantly by evidence of the world's lack of compassion. It's so hard to find kindness sometimes. How do you keep your chin up?

Although I try to keep a cheery exterior, I, too, occasionally get discouraged by the sheer magnitude of sadness and suffering around us, which, for the most part, has been caused by our own species. In addition, I have had my own share of personal challenges and sorrows, which, at times, have tested my optimism and outlook. Through my experiences, though, I have come to realize that each of us can only work with one small piece of the puzzle at a time. If we try to take on all life's problems at once, or attempt to carry the weight of the world on our shoulders, we will be crushed by the pressure of bearing such a burden. Furthermore, if we believe that we can alter everything we find intolerable, we will eventually be swallowed up by our own sense of self-importance.

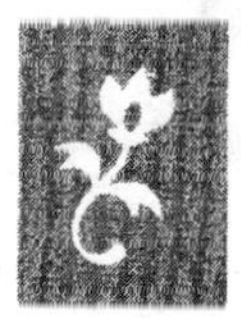

Veganism affords us a chance to live more fully and peacefully, knowing we are doing the best we can for those most in need.

My approach is one of trying to live in the moment, of compartmentalizing and doing what I can with what is right in front of me. What good is it if I try to save the world while ignoring the needs of someone close by, such as my spouse, a neighbor, or my animal companions? I also try to acknowledge and accept my shortcomings, knowing that as I become more tolerant of my own weaknesses, I will become more tolerant of others' as well. I have learned to laugh at myself and my foibles, and not take myself, my work, or my opinions too seriously.

As hard as it is sometimes, I endeavor to seek out the good in others and strive to live with conscious awareness. One of the ways I do this is by simply observing the inherent beauty that surrounds us but which so often gets overlooked–the sunrise and sunset, the soft breeze on my skin, the cloud formations, sunlight bouncing off leaves, a wild rabbit or squirrel. If I'm in my car sitting in traffic or stuck at a light, I use that time for quiet contemplation instead of getting impatient or angry and missing out on being alive at that instant.

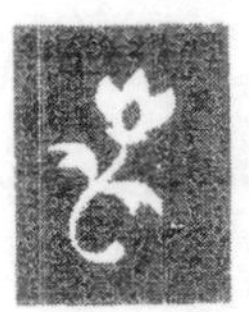

If we embody our ethics, the influence of our short presence on this earth will continue its effect long after we are gone.

The so-called negative day-to-day experiences, such as catching a cold, an appliance breaking, miserable weather, or other annoyances, are so inconsequential in light of more painful ordeals. I try to view these bad events as opportunities to learn and grow instead of fighting them, knowing that "this too shall pass."

It is not uncommon for vegans to become disheartened once in a while. Being keenly aware of the travails of others has its costs. But the benefits of being sensitive, caring, and cognizant of the struggles that most people turn their backs on affords us a chance to live more fully. There is an incredibly rewarding sense of peace and satisfaction in knowing that we are doing the best we can for those most in need. The outcome is irrelevant because, if we embody our ethics, the influence of our short presence on this earth will continue its effect long after we are gone. I do not delude myself by thinking I could personally turn the world upside down with my ideas; however, I fantasize that perhaps a few of them will stimulate others to try.

The little joys of life are what bring me pleasure and happiness. I keep my chin up by focusing on them and looking straight ahead–not up, down, around, or behind–just front, center, and always, always forward.

Mixed Relationships

I just recently started the process of going vegan and I am running into a problem with my wife. While she has no qualms about being vegetarian for her health, she thinks that being vegan is going too far and it's being radical. How should I deal with this?

There are many different reasons why people become vegetarian: religion and spirituality, ethics and compassion, health, the environment, finances, and hunger concerns, just to name a few. When people are drawn to vegetarianism for nonaltruistic purposes, such as improving their health, it is often hard for them to understand or appreciate what motivates others to veganism. Also, there is little incentive for them to extend their practice beyond diet. Conversely, when people choose vegetarianism for reasons outside themselves, they are able to view veganism as the next logical step.

Vegans challenge ingrained cultural assumptions that most of us have accepted since childhood, so it can be disquieting and at times difficult to be vegan. At every turn we are inculcated with slick, seductive marketing campaigns disseminated by governmental agencies, food-animal producers, and fast-food chains that have deep-seated financial interests in promoting particular commodities and perpetuating the benevolent myths we have about them. Questioning our cultural traditions and habits takes guts. Not only do vegans have to deal with making numerous personal adjustments, they must also confront the cynicism and scorn of suspicious friends and family members and a doubting public that doesn't want to be ruffled. It would be much easier to acquiesce to the status quo.

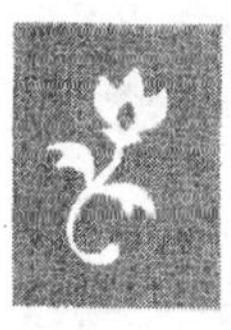

When people choose vegetarianism for reasons outside themselves, they are able to view veganism as the next logical step.

Nevertheless, vegans have a vision that is more profound than one driven by financial gain. Guided by compassion, vegans are willing to endure a few hassles in their mission to promote awareness of the cruelties and injustices our society overlooks or takes for granted. It is convenient for the public to classify vegans as rebels because vegan views are so drastically out of step with the mainstream. This does not imply that vegan beliefs are wrong—simply that they are different. There is nothing insurgent about embracing compassionate living. However, using products derived from cruelty when humane alternatives exist could most assuredly be construed as radical.

It is understandable that your wife is reluctant to become vegan. Few people would elect to go against the grain without a fervent belief in what they are doing. Unless your wife acknowledges the cruel realities behind the egg and dairy trades and recognizes the interconnectedness of the meat, dairy, and leather industries, she will have no impetus for being vegan. Just as a farmer plants fertile seeds but cannot make them sprout, you can deluge your wife with facts and figures but cannot penetrate her heart with them. She must be open, willing, and ready to comprehend the suffering that so moved you. Until that time, your choices will not make sense to her.

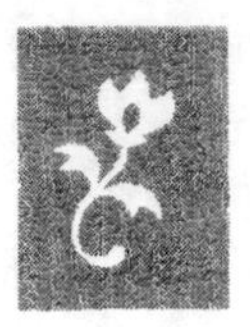

There is nothing insurgent about embracing compassionate living. However, using products derived from cruelty when humane alternatives exist could most assuredly be construed as radical.

It is hard to peel back the facade of the dairy, egg, and slaughter industries because their public persona is so widely sanitized and commercialized. Exposing oneself to the harsh truth can be painful, but it is necessary to live with honesty and a clear conscience.

It is invariably frustrating to be in a relationship where one person is highly committed to an ideal that the other person doesn't value or comprehend. Overcoming our cultural indoctrination and opening to veganism takes time. Many people who are now ardent vegans were once disbelievers. Your wife has already taken a giant step toward veganism by embracing a vegetarian diet, but it is quite possible this is as far as she may come. One of the deepest challenges of being vegan is respecting and honoring divergent viewpoints. Share with your wife the truth as you know it. Then love her enough to let her choose her own path.

My daughter, who is two years old, is a vegan, as am I. I have had no problems with her diet; however, her father is a meat-eater. He tried to be a vegetarian but broke down and was sneaking out to fast-food joints for burgers. He has a hard time understanding the reasons for being vegan. How can I convince him that my beliefs are valid?

A lasting marriage is a complex, intimate relationship between two people who are first and foremost best friends. The foundation of this friendship is built upon mutual trust and shared values. When one partner embraces drastically different ideals than those established at the outset of the marriage, such as becoming vegan, and the other does not, the relationship can become strained or threatened. When children are added to the mix, the problems are compounded.

Although people's values may progressively mature throughout their lifetime, they generally vary minimally. On the infrequent occasions when radical and abiding changes do occur, they are invariably predicated on evolving internal beliefs. That is, when people are awakened to the truth in their heart–not something learned intellectually or externally, but validated from within–they can be stimulated to reevaluate their ethics and actions. Without this inward realization, however, few people are persuaded to alter their core principles.

There is no way to force an individual to adopt someone else's moral code, no matter how righteous the motivation. You can supply your husband with all the information about veganism he can absorb, but that doesn't necessarily mean you will render a permanent shift in his perspective. His heart must first be open to the reality that inspires people to the vegan way of life. Without an open heart, no amount of facts or figures can influence him.

Nevertheless, you can help your husband to understand your own motivations by sharing books, magazines, pamphlets, and videos with him. These can assist you in conveying to your husband your personal impetus for being vegan, but do not use them to pressure him to "see things your way." If you push him, he may very well reject whatever you ask of him and shut you out. The fact that he would go out to get a burger without telling you is evidence that he doesn't feel safe enough to be open about his divergent opinions.

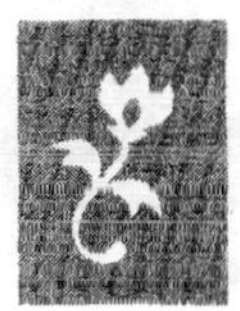

Only when people are awakened to the truth in their heart—not something learned intellectually or externally, but validated from within—can they be stimulated to reevaluate their ethics and actions.

For a marriage to endure, both parties must feel sufficiently comfortable in their own home to let their guard down and be themselves. It is vital that you both come to terms with your differences so you can relax and speak honestly in each other's presence. Let your husband know how significant veganism is to you as an individual and as a mother. Then let him have equal time to express his viewpoint. Remember that he will be candid only if he feels he will be heard without judgment.

It takes courage and tolerance to remain in a "mixed marriage" and to respectfully determine how to handle the matters of everyday life. There will be many decisions ahead of you, not the least of which are those surrounding the raising of your daughter.

Parents need to present a unified value system to their children. Therefore, you and your husband must come to an agreement about some very basic issues. Will your husband comply with and support your decision to raise your daughter vegan? How will you instill in your daughter the fundamental ethics of veganism while providing a way for her to honor her father's differences? Can you concur on what food choices are appropriate? Are you able to present a united position to grandparents and other relatives? Are you both prepared to explain to family members, friends' parents, and teachers what food, toys, clothing, and personal care items are or are not acceptable and why?

Then there are personal issues. What is your comfort level regarding your husband purchasing nonvegan items, such as leather products, and bringing them into the home? Could you tolerate him cooking meat at home, perhaps in the same pans you might use to prepare a vegan dish? How do feel about him eating meat or dairy products in front of your daughter? How will you handle having company over for dinner or going out to eat? Can you trust that your husband will not offer your daughter meat or dairy products when the two of them are out of your presence?

These are profound concerns that can penetrate the nucleus of your marriage. You each have much soul searching and inner exploring to do before you can both feel reassured that your separate points of view will be reciprocally respected and valued. Nevertheless, try to begin the process as soon as possible, because there are several entities at stake: your daughter, your husband, yourself, your marriage, and your family.

I became vegan during my relationship with my partner. He does not feel as strongly as I do, and it is really taking a toll on me. He eats mostly vegetarian but continues to buy meat for his son. He also wears leather clothes and shoes, silk ties, and so on. I feel disempowered and sacrificial, being unable to set the boundary of not having animal products in my home. This really seems to have altered the unified parental structure that I feel is necessary. My respect for myself and him is diminishing. After a year of trying to be open, I'm not feeling any sense of peace.

The sense of frustration and isolation you are experiencing within your relationship is apparent. It is challenging enough for vegans to be out of step with the culture at large, but to feel alienated within your own home is especially difficult.

It is important to continue to communicate with your partner and not distance yourself further because of your feelings. Be honest and open without letting your emotions cloud what you need to say. Give him the space to share his point of view, too, without reproach. Be sure to include your concerns about his son and about maintaining a unified parental approach, as well as about your desire to uphold a vegan household.

Even though the situation may seem bleak at the moment, remember that your partner is nearly vegetarian, and that's already a major step in the vegan direction. If his motivation for eating a mostly vegetarian diet is because of pressure from you or because of his own health concerns, you may want to supply him with some basic vegan literature so he can read about other issues with which he may not be familiar. Also give him information on the soundness of a vegan diet for children, since he is probably purchasing meat because he is convinced his son needs it to thrive. Be sure the materials you present have been written by professionals such as physicians or dietitians, so he can rest assured that the information is scientific rather than biased.

As with most personal revelations, vegans are usually eager to share their new awareness with those they care about most. It can be incredibly disappointing to realize that our loved ones may not be as excited as we are, or sometimes may not even be interested. Allowing your partner the freedom to progress at his own rate may be one of the greatest tests of your willingness to be sensitive and empathic toward those who hold differing beliefs.

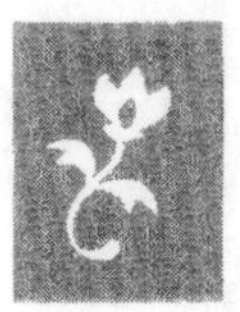

Most people who come to veganism feel jolted awake, as though they had been asleep at the wheel and are only now becoming conscious of the truth that has always surrounded them.

In the midst of even the most ordinary relationship conflicts, it is easy to denounce the other person entirely. In other words, we might think of them as *completely* irrational, *totally* unreasonable, *always* inflexible, or *perpetually* stubborn. During times of turmoil, it's much easier to see our "opposition" in terms of black and white, all or nothing, while discounting the more worthy qualities that drew us toward that person in the first place. Often these attributes are perfectly intact, just much less visible through the foggy lens of friction.

Recall what you most admire and love about your partner and focus on these special qualities when you are together and apart. Tell him how important and special he is to you, and how meaningful it would be to share the commitment of veganism. Try to remember what you were like before you became vegan and know that your partner is simply at the place where you once were.

If you feel that your desire to have a more complete vegan lifestyle outweighs your tolerance, patience, and love for your partner, then you will need to make the difficult decision to separate. Only you can ascertain the level of dissatisfaction and unrest you can endure. After discussing the matter with your partner, determine what you must do to regain consonance in your heart and your home. Whatever direction you choose, engender it with tenderness and respect for your partner, his son, and yourself. Be an example of vegan compassion through loving actions and words. Then, regardless of what you decide, peace and serenity will follow.

How do I convert a barbecuing, meat-loving, tough Army guy, or should I even try? Even more important—how do I convince him that any children we may be blessed with should be raised as vegans? Won't it confuse them if Mom is a vegan and Dad eats meat?

More than passion, similar backgrounds, common interests, outlook, or goals, abiding relationships depend on shared values to ensure success. Veganism is as important as any other conviction and perhaps even more so, because vegan practice encompasses virtually every aspect of daily living. From meals to clothing, from entertainment to occupation, few moments pass in a day when vegans aren't reminded of their beliefs. Consequently, vegans can feel very lonely in a mixed relationship, even within their own home, which, for most people, is the one place they can take solace from an often hostile world.

There is no way to convert anyone to veganism. Some people can be exposed to all the horror, gore, and irrefutable facts about animal suffering and slaughter and not even wince. Those who embrace veganism must first be open to growing, learning, and changing, not just intellectually but emotionally, philosophically, and spiritually. This is not a process that can be forced. People who adopt a lasting vegan lifestyle do so only when they are ready, not at a time their partner dictates, and must proceed at their own pace. If the head is willing but the heart is closed, veganism will simply be a temporary exercise in self-denial. It won't endure because there is no compelling reason to persevere. In such cases, veganism is merely a way to quiet a nagging companion.

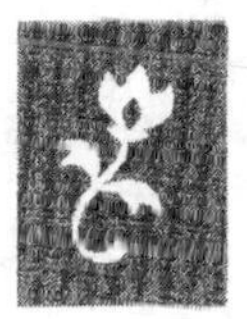

Those who embrace veganism must first be open to growing, learning, and changing. If the head is willing but the heart is closed, veganism will simply be a temporary exercise in self-denial.

If a couple cannot see eye-to eye on the essentials of their joint lives, it will be virtually impossible to raise children with a clear and unwavering value system. At its core, veganism is about making right choices. If Mom is right, then Dad must be wrong–there is no practical way to achieve full balance in such a situation. Effective coparenting requires the adults to present a unified stance. Each must model the behavior they expect of their children. It is confusing for children to be forced to decide which parental example should be followed. In a mixed relationship, children are obliged to take sides. That is an unfair position in which to place a youngster.

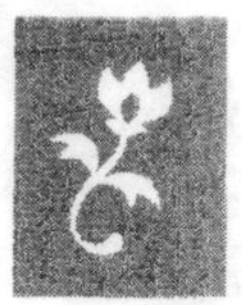

Effective coparenting requires the adults to present a unified stance and model the behavior they expect of their children.

Now—long before you have offspring—is the time to evaluate your relationship, prioritize what is important to you and determine which concessions you are and are not willing to make. The Army is not conducive to a vegan lifestyle and such a decision might complicate matters for your partner and his career. Nonetheless, you cannot second-guess his choices. Give him a chance. Talk to him and openly discuss your worries, hopes, and dreams. Together you may be able to devise a plan for your shared future that meets the expectations and goals you both have. He may even be more amenable to veganism than you anticipate.

A relationship is a two-way street. Although your concerns are valid, they will remain hypothetical until they are brought out into the open and examined within the context of the loving trust you and your partner have established.

I have been vegan for a few months, after being an ovolacto vegetarian for eleven years. My boyfriend of four years eats meat, loves cheese, cream sauces, and other dairy-rich foods and is not fond of fresh fruits and vegetables. He has eaten soy cheeses and meat substitutes but still prefers the real thing. This makes having meals together very difficult! How can we bring our eating habits more in synch with each other?

For most people, sharing food with those we love is an act of nurturing and an expression of unity. At the same time, food choices are very personal. Everyone's preferences differ, and what excites one person may be unpalatable to another.

Because vegan values extend beyond the palate and the plate, vegans who do not like particular foods will seek out alternatives to meet their nutritional needs and satisfy their tastes. For vegans, eliminating the products of animal suffering from their diet and lives is a matter of conscience, not an issue of denial or inconvenience. This is what can make living with a nonvegan so exasperating.

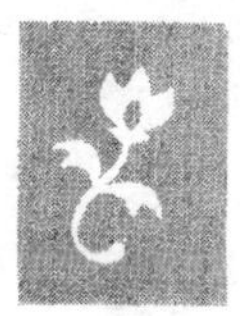

For vegans, eliminating the products of suffering from their diet and lives is a matter of conscience, not an issue of denial or inconvenience.

Because food has been such a point of contention for both of you, it is important to jointly devise some guidelines that you each can accept. For instance, you may not want to purchase or cook meat for your boyfriend but would agree to him buying and cooking it for himself. Or, you may feel that having meat in your home is intolerable, but you would agree to him eating meat out of the house. You could decide that when you go out to eat you will select a restaurant that serves both vegetarian and nonvegetarian dishes, and so on.

Bear in mind that transitioning to new flavors and textures in food can be emotionally taxing, and giving up foods that one has loved since childhood can feel like a tangible loss. Try preparing dishes that are commonplace but not considered strictly vegetarian, for example, bean burritos, spaghetti with marinara sauce, baked potatoes, baked beans, stir-fries, a hearty soup or stew, vegan pancakes, or vinaigrette potato salad. If you make dishes that are familiar and delicious in their own right and are not necessarily substitutes for anything, your boyfriend may find them more appealing, because he's not comparing them with their meat or dairy counterpart.

Acknowledge that you may never come to a full agreement on the issue of food, and realize that employing tolerance and acceptance may be the only way to preserve your relationship. If you extend your love and compassion to him without coercion or condemnation, you may one day find his heart opening in directions you never imagined.

Raising Vegan Children

I am raising my two children (one age four years and the other eight months) vegan. Now that my four-year-old is "out in the world," I am coming up against so many difficult ethical issues involving his fitting in while adhering to a vegan lifestyle. For instance, today his little friend was visiting and wanted to pretend to fish. I told his friend

I didn't like fishing because it hurt and killed the fish. My little boy looked at me as if he were embarrassed, even though when we are alone together he believes in animal rights and even asks me to read animal rescue stories, including articles on why fishing is just as bad as hunting. I don't know if I should simply take a back seat and let him feel that he's fitting in by "pretending," as he told me he was doing in front of his friend, or if I should be more didactic about it and not allow it. This is one isolated incident among many that come up every day. Do you have any suggestions?

It is difficult, if not impossible, to control all the stimuli to which children are exposed. The best that parents can do is to provide constructive verbal guidance and congruous role modeling that reinforce their beliefs. Children become confused, frustrated, and angry when parents say one thing and do another. Maintaining consistency between what you tell your children and your own behavior will provide a powerful paradigm of the vegan beliefs you wish to instill.

Most parents want their offspring to adopt values similar to their own, but the only way this transfer will occur is if parents are directly involved in their children's lives. Positive and negative beliefs and behaviors are fostered chiefly by one technique—example. Even when we aren't conscious of it, children are watching and digesting our every move. To credibly convey your vegan convictions to your children, they must be a part of all your interactions with them.

You cannot regulate what transpires outside your home, but within it you can establish clear standards of conduct regarding what is and isn't acceptable. When it comes to setting limits, people both young and old respond more readily if they are personally involved than if there is autocratic control. When children know why their parents believe and act as they do, it is easier for them to appreciate and accept their values as their own. This is key if your children are to maintain their vegan ethics when they are away from you, in challenging situations, or among antagonistic peers or adults. Their veganism must belong to them and be embraced by them for them to sustain it.

If certain types of play are unacceptable to you, discourage them. For instance, if you find toy guns offensive because you do not want your children to act out their play in real life, or if you believe pretend violence is a potential precursor to actual violence, then prohibiting toy guns or cruel games is reasonable. The same can be said of activities that simulate harming or killing animals, regardless of the intention. To help young children comprehend the motivation behind your restrictions, offer a brief but lucid explanation; then guide them to alternative activities that are equally engaging but more humane.

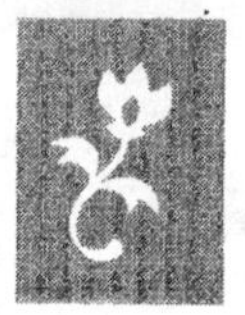

When children know why their parents believe and act as they do, it is easier for them to appreciate and accept their values as their own.

Although you detected embarrassment in your son, it may have been your own emotions, facial expressions, or tone of voice being reflected back to you through your son's reaction. At this age, his response in these situations is most likely based on the impressions he picks up directly from you rather than on a true feeling of chagrin. If you are proud of and secure in your vegan ethics, your children will sense this and will radiate their own confidence and high self-esteem about being vegan.

As a vegan parent, you can only hope that your children will aspire to a compassionate way of life, but there are no guarantees. If you offer them the empathy, understanding, and respect you ask of them, and provide a loving example of your principles in action, your children will have an ideal teacher and you will have the greatest likelihood of success.

My husband and I are strict vegans. Our two kids—ages four and seven—have recently decided to be ovolacto vegetarians. They love animals and vow not to eat them, but ice cream and cheese pizza are another thing! I've tried the vegan counterparts, but they refuse to eat them. What's a vegan mom to do?

When children are young, they depend on their parents to make all the important decisions for them. In most circumstances, children are incapable of determining what is in their best interests, so parents must intervene. In particular, this includes issues of safety and health, but parents also intercede on matters of morality, respect, courtesy, and social convention. We have an obligation to our children to protect them from harm. In addition, we have a responsibility to prevent them from harming others. Children learn not only by the example we present to them but from the parameters we set for them as well.

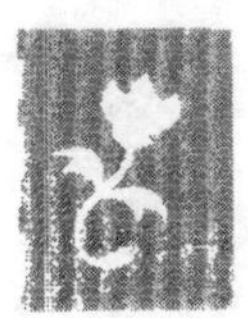

Children learn not only by the examples we present but from the parameters we set for them.

Veganism is no different from any other moral guideline that parents establish for their children. There are many behaviors that parents simply would not tolerate from their children, other children, or even adult guests in their home. Now is the time for your kids to develop the beliefs and habits you want them to adopt for a lifetime. Peer pressure and social conformation should have nothing to do with the standards you determine for your children. There are countless demands your little ones could make that you would not cave in on. If vegan principles are important for you to instill in your children, then now is the time to activate them.

I recently became vegan and am raising my little boy to respect our fellow creatures. I can't tell you the criticism I get in his school, as if I'm abusing my son because he doesn't eat flesh. I bring literature to his teachers, but they don't seem to have an open mind and they never comment on it. This year Thanksgiving was extremely difficult for us because his school had a party and children all around him were eating meat. One of the visiting teachers leaned over to him with a chicken leg and my son told her, "I don't eat animals." I was so proud of him, even though I'm sure it was stressful. Do you have any suggestions about dealing with my son and his teachers? I know he feels good about being vegan, but I just hope it stays that way.

No doubt about it, raising a vegan child in our very nonvegan world is a difficult task. It does take extra thought, care, and planning, especially in environments where there are no other vegans. Holidays are a special challenge for both vegan parents and their children because there are countless cultural practices and assumptions that clash with vegan beliefs, and there is a lot of pressure from nonvegan teachers, friends, family, and other parents to conform.

Because your son is so young and he is enrolled in a mainstream school environment, your continued involvement is essential. The teachers do not need to know or understand the rationale behind your beliefs, and it is perhaps unreasonable to presume that they would show any more than a perfunctory interest. What matters is that they are aware of, respect, and comply with your wishes and ensure that your son is not picked on, bullied, shamed, pitied, or ridiculed for being different. They should not draw attention to him because he is vegan but, instead, help him fit in with his other schoolmates. It is also crucial that your son's teacher provides alternative snacks whenever the rest of the students are given treats that contain animal products, just as she would do if there were a student who keeps kosher or one who is allergic to certain foods. His teacher must be made aware that you and your son celebrate some holidays in alternative ways, and this should be regarded no less significantly than any religious or cultural difference.

It is unreasonable to expect your son's teacher to know much about veganism or care much about it, as this may be her very first exposure. She may not always remember to advise a visiting teacher or aide about your son's needs, which is why your ongoing presence may be needed. It is your responsibility to remind the teacher about your son's veganism shortly before upcoming events or special occasions and perhaps discuss options for him or provide suggestions. If you are in attendance at special programs or parties held at the school, it would be a good idea for you to personally inform the guest teachers and aides that your son does not eat animal products and that they should not offer any to him.

Teachers should ensure that vegan students are not picked on, bullied, shamed, pitied, or ridiculed for being different.

It is impractical to anticipate that your son's teacher would adapt the curriculum, story telling, or free play to reflect a vegan or pro-animal theme. Consequently, you may want to make some recommendations regarding reading material and games. In addition, it would be a good idea to have a heart-to-heart talk with the teacher about your concerns. The more forthright you are the better. The teacher cannot surmise your hopes or standards or your son's needs, so it is up to you to explain, propose ideas, and offer solutions.

As long as your son is in a mixed environment, he is going to run into similar situations. While he is young, he depends on you to provide direct support. At this age, he should never be put in the awkward position of having to defend his veganism. In time, he will learn from your loving intervention and strong vegan example how to respond respectfully and intelligently in tough circumstances like this. Then, when he is a little older, he will be empowered to feel comfortable, confident, and proud anywhere he goes because he will be secure about who he is and in what he believes.

My sixteen-year-old daughter went to town last evening to eat out with kids from our community youth group. She ordered a vegan entrée, and when her meal arrived, the other children started mocking and insulting her by saying how disgusting her meal choice was. The adult leaders of the group just sat at the other end of the table and smiled. I am disturbed and embarrassed about the way the adults handled this, and I am so disappointed in those kids! I plan on telling the leaders that my daughter says she probably will never go out to eat with the group again.

It sounds like you've raised a very courageous individual who is not afraid to stand by her convictions. In the teen milieu, where conformity reigns supreme, it takes guts to be unconventional. It is sad, however, that many adults do not share her pluck and determination and are willing to sacrifice principles for popularity. Their behavior reflects the attitude of many young people and sets a flawed and dangerous precedent. As a culture, we expect adults to act maturely and be positive, nurturing role models for our youth. We also presume that as interim guardians they will protect our children and respond to them with respect and compassion. Unfortunately, there is no guarantee that adults will behave less like juveniles than their charges.

Your decision to approach the youth group leaders is a sensible one. It is up to parents to explain their children's special requirements to any adults who will have temporary custody of them. Based on this particular incident, it is also important for you to express your desire for the leaders to help make your daughter feel a part of the group and not be singled out for her differences.

Young people can be particularly cruel in their teasing, and what may seem malicious to one person could be interpreted as ordinary adolescent behavior to another. It is possible that the adults did not consider the episode especially vicious, even though your daughter clearly felt rejected and picked on. The truth of the circumstance is irrelevant. What matters is that she had a dreadful experience to which the group leaders were either blind or insensitive.

No young person should be forced to sacrifice participation in a group because the adults in command are oblivious. Approach the group leaders with empathy, knowing that they may be unaware of the ethical underpinnings surrounding your daughter's food choices. Try to be sensitive to the fact that they, like the young people involved, are seeking the group's approval and may be concerned that if they had defended your daughter they might have sacrificed their own acceptance with the kids. This, of course, does not exonerate their behavior, nor does it justify ignoring your daughter's apparent need for assistance and support. The adults should be held culpable for this pained situation, be willing to make amends by apologizing, and devise a policy of intervention so this will not happen to any participant in this group again.

Adults in leadership roles have a responsibility to teach and be examples of tolerance. It is a parent's role to ensure that the adults in their children's lives fulfill this duty. Parents should never allow the taunting of their children–or anyone else's–because their skin color, religion, culture, aptitude, or physical challenges make them unique among their peers. Veganism is no different in this regard. It deserves the same compliant understanding and deference.

Dealing with Parents

I am a fifteen-year-old vegan living in a household of meat-eaters. My mother won't accept that I don't eat animal products and won't let me make my own meals. How do I convince her that I am perfectly able to make nutritious vegan meals? I can't live on bread and veggies forever!

You are in a very challenging predicament and your heartache is evident. It is difficult to be a teen with strong convictions, especially when no one seems to take your viewpoints seriously.

You are entitled to your beliefs. They are important and deserve respect, regardless of your age. Unfortunately, age can be a barrier to personal freedom and individuality within a household. Typically, it is the adults who pay the bills, set the rules, and have the final say. When parents balk at a daughter or son's decision to become vegan, it is often due to one or more factors. Here are just a few possibilities:

- Your mother may not know very much about veganism. She may be embarrassed to admit that she doesn't have a clue about what to cook or how to plan meals for you, and she may be unaware about where to get information.
- Your mother may have read misleading stories that present vegan diets as extreme or radical.
- Your mother may have heard that teenage girls with eating disorders or a fear of getting fat sometimes use veganism as a way to control their weight.
- Your mother may believe this is just a phase that you will outgrow.
- Your mother may think you are unable to prepare nutritious meals based on her observation of your past cooking experiences, food choices, or eating habits.
- Your mother may be hurt that you won't eat the food she prepares and could be angry about being pressured to make something different just for you.

- Your mother may be troubled about the extra cost of buying special foods.

Talk to your mother and candidly express your reasons for wanting to be vegan, without going into unnecessary detail or graphic explanations. Let her know that this is exceedingly important to you and how much her help and support would mean to you. Stay calm and be receptive to your mother's point of view without caving in about your own. Do some research ahead of time to familiarize yourself with vegan nutrition and meal planning for teens. If you approach the discussion with maturity and sensitivity to your mother's concerns, you should be able to work out a solution that will appease her while accommodating your beliefs.

Remember that you are in control of your own body and what you put into it should ultimately be your decision. No one can force you to eat certain foods, but it is essential that you get sufficient nutrition. Avoid being hostile toward your mother even if she does not concede. Anger will only damage your spirit and hurt your relationship. If you demonstrate personal responsibility and show appreciation for your mother's effort and concerns, she may very well come around in time.

As a vegan, I go through a lot of hassles with my dad. He has no sympathy for the suffering of animals. He does not believe that a vegan diet is healthier than a meat-based one. He thinks that the brain can only function correctly when it has animal protein. He also believes that we need meat to be strong, have energy, and learn. How can I prove to him that he is wrong?

Many people are misinformed about veganism or know very little about it. What we don't know can seem frightening and threatening and may cause us to be skeptical or defensive. This is especially true for issues related to diet.

There is no point in trying to prove that your father is wrong and you are right. This will only result in a futile battle of the wills and a lot of useless anger, neither of which will draw you closer or make you respect each other more. The vegan tenets of doing the least harm and eliminating suffering include you and your father as well.

You cannot change your father's mind and force him to have sympathy for animals. Compassion begins in the heart. If your father's heart is not open to this notion, thrusting it upon him will only breed indignation and resentment. Actually, it is not necessary that you and your father agree on this issue as long as you honor each other's right to have separate points of view. Neither of you needs to acquiesce to the other's position in order to maintain your individual convictions.

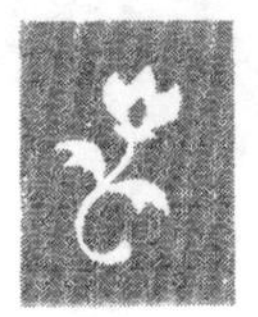

Demonstrating grace toward those who give us the hardest time can be one of the toughest challenges of being vegan.

It is irrelevant whether a vegan or omnivorous diet is more healthful. The truth is, a person can be well or ill following either one. Many factors are associated with physical fitness, and diet is only one of them. A vegan can have very poor eating habits, as can an omnivore. It is unfair to promote the belief that all vegans are inherently healthy (or at least healthier than omnivores), because it is not necessarily true. Vegans suffer from genetic disorders, environmental hazards, and acquired diseases the same as the general public. However, a well-balanced plant-based diet along with other healthful lifestyle practices provides some protective benefits in ways that the standard meat-centered diet cannot.

But what if a vegan diet had no health benefits whatsoever? Would you still subscribe to a life of dynamic harmlessness? My guess is that you would, and that is the bottom line. The issue, then, is less about veganism being better than it is about simply being a healthful and ethical alternative.

For your father to accept your choice, you need to exhibit a mature approach. This involves acknowledging your dad's concern for your well-being by demonstrating that you are capable of devising and following a well-balanced vegan diet based on current nutritional guidelines. It includes buying your own food and being willing to prepare your own meals, if necessary, without complaining. It also means that you can restore harmony and let your dad save face by refraining from trying to prove him wrong. Even though your father believes that meat is necessary for optimum mental and physical functioning, he will realize on his own that he is mistaken if you are well nourished, stay fit, and excel in your schoolwork and extracurricular activities. This will take some effort on your part, but seeing is believing. Nothing will convince your dad more that veganism is rational and sound than the example of your own glowing health and personal accomplishments.

I am fifteen years old and my beliefs and who I am as a person are not respected or even acknowledged by my family. Instead, they are considered laughing matters and walked all over. How much of a problem could they have with being happy for me for my decision to be vegan and help animals? I don't understand them, they don't understand me, and I don't think there will ever be understanding between us.

Most parents love their children and want them to be successful and happy. Often this means helping their children to fit in and conform to cultural standards. When parents discourage their children from unconventional behavior, it is usually because they don't want to see them suffer the social consequences of "being different."

Many parents are ill equipped to cope with the challenges that face young adults today, and they may have difficulty accepting that their children have a mind of their own. This can be especially painful for parents if their children's perspectives are the complete opposite of theirs. It often seems easier to criticize kids than to take a serious look at what they are saying. Adults can be intimidated by the contrary views of their children that provoke them to carefully evaluate their own belief system. This is because if they don't like what they uncover, they may feel obligated to change, and change is an unappealing nuisance for most of us. Broadly speaking, parents don't like to have their values examined; they just want their children to embrace them without question.

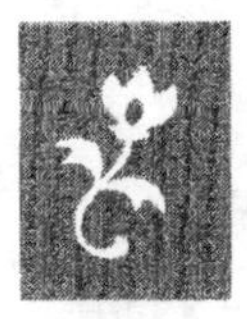

Adults can be intimidated by the contrary views of their children that provoke them to carefully evaluate their own belief system.

Just like you, your parents hurt, have fears, and want approval, and chances are that your conflicting views are driving them up a wall. This is not your fault, of course, and you should not feel guilty or obligated to change who you are simply because your parents–or anyone else–don't like or approve of your ideals. Bear in mind that ridicule is just one way that people lash out when they are feeling frustrated.

Anger is like an image in a mirror—it is always reflected right back at us.

Getting angry at your parents for being who they are is tantamount to them getting angry at you for who you are. It is pointless. There is no need for them to understand your beliefs for you to get along and respect each other. You can still maintain your vegan practices even if your parents do not fully appreciate the motivation behind them. Try to keep your cool when you tell them what you will and will not eat or do. You can explain if they ask or are interested. Otherwise, simply set the parameters for your own behavior and then let the issue go.

Attempt to look at the situation from your parents' point of view. Even though this won't be easy, you are asking the same of them. Try to have empathy for them, because they don't know any other way to respond to you or your veganism. Remind yourself that in a few short years you will be able to engage your principles completely, and realize that anger and intolerance are no more vegan than eating meat or wearing leather. When the sarcastic comments and mockery come flying in your direction, remind yourself how wonderful you really are and how lucky you are to have become aware of compassion at such an early age. Keep your heart and your mind open. Instead of letting the harsh words stick in you like a knife, let them float through you, as if you were pure light and the words were only air. Be proud of how you respond as you take the vegan high road. Know that the tough times you face now will empower you to be a stronger, wiser, and more merciful adult.

I decided to be a vegetarian about six months ago and have not touched meat since then. I recently chose not to eat eggs or cheese, yet I still drink milk, making me not a vegan. The members of my family don't understand my reasons for my lifestyle. They think it's stupid. My father always teases me, my mother very seldom remembers that I don't eat fish (according to her, fish isn't meat), and my sisters are always asking if I'd mind eating meat for one day so we can go to a steakhouse. My family is going to visit our relatives in a different country soon, and I will be living with them for two months. I will be surrounded by a bunch of people who oppose my choice and I'll be asked a million questions a day (even more than I get asked now, which is sometimes more than I can handle). Please help me to deal with this!

When young people adopt beliefs that are contrary to their family's customs, it is not unusual for there to be resistance. When that choice is vegetarianism, and there was no previous hint that such a change was on the horizon, parents are taken by surprise.

If you never told your family that you were even thinking about becoming a vegetarian, there is no way they could be prepared for such news. Therefore, they may presume that you are just experimenting and that your choice is temporary. Most people know very little about vegetarianism, except for distorted impressions advanced by ill-informed media. Considering the myths that are circulated about vegetarianism, your parents cannot be faulted for their mistaken assertion that "fish isn't meat."

Because you are the person who initiated the change, the brunt of educating your family falls on your shoulders. However, before you can enlighten others, you must grasp the issues thoroughly yourself and understand what motivates you to be a vegetarian.

You mentioned that you recently stopped eating eggs and cheese but continue to drink cow's milk. Are you in transition to becoming a vegan? If so, your family may not understand the reasoning behind what could appear to them to be a sudden and drastic transformation. If your impetus is an ethic of compassion, be aware that others will probably comment on the inconsistency of not eating cheese but drinking milk. Although for many people the progression to veganism is gradual, outsiders may expect an overnight metamorphosis, and they are often quick to point out moral inconsistencies. Have you examined your reasons for giving up some but not all animal products? Have you considered the connection between other commodities and animal suffering? Are you clear about the path you have chosen, why it is important to you, and how you intend to pursue it?

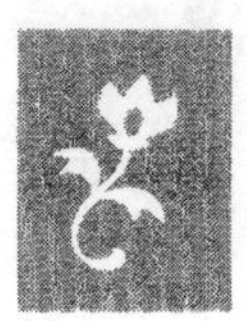

Although for many people the progression to veganism is gradual, outsiders may expect an overnight metamorphosis, and they are often quick to point out moral inconsistencies.

As long as you fully comprehend what compels you to be vegan or vegetarian, you will be prepared to deal honestly and respectfully with the flurry of questions and remarks your relatives toss your way. You will also be better equipped to maintain your commitment in foreign surroundings where vegetarian options may be limited.

There is no point in getting indignant about your family's misinformation and insensitivity. It is reasonable to assume that their barbs are innocent and stem from their loving concern about your well-being. Your parents may also be worried that as a vegetarian you won't be able to fully participate in family functions or other social activities. Your father's teasing may simply be a way for him to gently vent his tension, or it could be a playful attempt to stay close with you. Try to laugh along with him. Learning to take yourself and your family's razzing less seriously will go a long way in tempering the strain of your present relationship.

Once your own feelings are sorted out, talk to your family and let them know that you have given this matter much thought and would be grateful for their help and respect. If you approach them with the deference you hope to receive, it is more likely to be reciprocated. Once they realize that you are informed and sincere about your decision, they'll be better equipped to support you at home and during your travels. Self-inquiry will help you better understand your convictions and will bring about greater determination and self-confidence, qualities that will be apparent whether you're expressing your ideas to family, friends, or strangers.

I have spent my entire adult life bouncing between vegetarianism and macrobiotics. This past year was definitive for me because I finally dropped fish from my diet and several months ago dropped dairy and eggs and started my journey toward veganism. I became more educated about the suffering of animals and felt my lifestyle changes were beneficial to all living creatures. It was a personal triumph! However, my family (particularly my mother) and some friends are adamant that I am ruining my health and that this must be just a fad or phase. My mother is taking my choice personally. How can I convince her that she raised an intelligent, caring, and productive member of society?

When people adopt a diet or lifestyle that is radically different from what their friends and family follow, it can be disconcerting for everyone involved. Friends may feel betrayed; parents may feel forsaken; and all parties could easily become defensive.

Now that you have chosen the vegan path, your loved ones may feel they can no longer participate in your life or share meaningful activities with you. They may believe you have renounced their values, which, in part, is probably true. Consequently, they may feel hurt and angry. Those near to you may imagine you are judging them, which could make them even more suspicious of your intent. The natural tendency to safeguard habits could further provoke your friends and family to question your sincerity and attempt to dissuade you or prove you wrong.

Many new vegans experience a similar backlash. Even though veganism is gaining wider recognition and broader acceptance, it is still far to the left of the mainstream. No matter what your individual approach or perspective, vegan practice rattles the status quo.

Beyond the apparent resistance, however, is likely a genuine concern for your well-being. Your mother's generation was raised with certain notions about which foods are vital to maintain good health. After a lifetime of indoctrination, these assumptions have become deeply ingrained and are very difficult to dislodge. In addition to inferring that her parental wisdom has been challenged, it is not surprising that your mother has concluded your health will decline if you don't eat the way that she does.

Gaining your family and friends' acceptance will take time and patience. They may never fully appreciate your personal triumph, of which you should feel quite proud. Nor may they understand what sparked your decision to become vegan. They may always think that you are just going through a fad or phase, even after years of being vegan.

You are the same wonderful person you were before you became vegan. If your family and friends didn't perceive your splendid attributes previously, it is doubtful they will notice them now. From their point of view, the fact that you are vegan may only obscure your virtues further. On the other hand, if your loved ones have always appreciated your special qualities, being vegan should not eclipse their view. In time, through your own tolerance and loving example, they may come to realize that your principled way of life does not detract from who you are or have been. It is merely another extension of your already established compassionate nature.

I would like to see my late-middle-aged parents consume a healthier diet. I have been stocking their refrigerator and freezer with easy-to-prepare entrées and meat alternatives, but my enthusiasm doesn't seem to be catching on. Am I being overzealous or is there a better way of convincing my parents that "this vegetarianism" is not only more healthful for them but would be easier on their pocketbook and better for the environment?

Wanting your parents to live as long and healthfully as possible is unquestionably a noble ideal. It is also very considerate of you to make it easier for them to adopt a vegetarian diet by providing handy foods that require minimal preparation. Despite your fervor and thoughtfulness, there are probably several reasons why your parents are not equally jubilant about the idea of becoming vegetarians.

Your vegetarianism was a personal choice. No one strong-armed you into making that decision, so you remained in control of when and how you transitioned to it. You had your own reasons for electing to become a vegetarian, which most likely provided inspiration and support for you. Because you were in charge of your destiny, you could be proud of your journey as well as your arrival.

All individuals want that same sense of command over their lives. When others tell us what we ought to do, it is infuriating—especially when they think they know what is best for us or believe they know us better than we know ourselves. Regulating other people's lives, even when it appears to be in their best interests, can erode self-esteem and threaten autonomy.

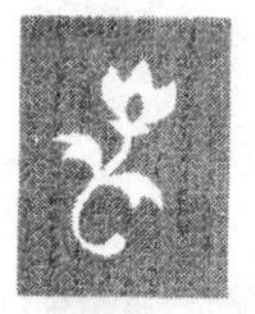

Everyone must find her or his own incentive to change. It won't come from somebody else; it will happen from within.

Food is an especially delicate point of contention because it represents more than just a way to quell our appetite and nourish our bodies. For a lot of people, food is a way to nurture and indulge an even deeper hunger—our emotional desire for love and security. Furthermore, food can represent our ethnicity, upbringing, and cultural heritage. It can be nostalgic, consoling, or celebratory. So, when we encourage others to change their diet, it is a more profound request than might appear on the surface.

Oddly enough, people tend to recoil most when those with whom they are closest try to influence them to change. When it comes to diet, outsiders often garner greater respect and attention. Perhaps it is because they are unbiased and detached, making them appear more credible. This could be yet another reason why your parents tune out what you tell them about vegetarianism. Sometimes books, pamphlets, and brochures are more persuasive than one-on-one conversations with loved ones.

Another possible factor in your parents' indifference could be their unfamiliarity with vegetarian cuisine. We all have our own unique tastes and, for some of us, new foods can be nothing short of frightening. Maybe the items you've selected are not the types of foods they prefer. You could ask them to suggest alternatives if they don't like what you picked out, but they may not have any idea what options are available. One way around this would be for you to cook dinner for your parents occasionally so they could sample a few new foods. You could even devise a buffet of various frozen entrées so they would have a chance to test them before you make future purchases.

You are a very special person to actively care so much about your parents' well-being. If your parents do not respond to your loving efforts, it doesn't mean that you have failed. They may just not be ready or interested enough to hear your message. Try to give your parents enough space and respect to make up their own minds about what they should eat. Evidently that's what they did for you, and you certainly made excellent choices.

Family Values

Last year my ten-year-old niece asked me why I didn't want any turkey for Thanksgiving. My brother-in-law explained to her that I was a vegetarian. Since then, it's rare that my niece will eat meat, and if she doesn't want anything my sister made for dinner, she'll simply say, "Sorry, Mommy, but that's meat—I'm a vegetarian, just like Auntie." Needless to say, my sister is quite upset with me. Every time I've been alone with my niece she has asked if I am still a vegetarian. I always tell her yes, and she says, "Me too!" Now that I have become vegan, my sister has told me not to tell my niece or even let her know what *vegan* means. I think that's wrong but, since she's not my child, I feel obligated to follow my sister's wishes. I am proud of being vegan and don't want to hide this part of me from my niece—it would feel as if I were lying about who I am! My niece looks up to me and cares deeply about animals. I want to encourage her feelings of compassion but I don't want to make my sister angry.

No one should feel compelled to conceal her or his identity just because someone else is ill equipped to cope with it. Veganism is the sum of a person's character. It is not a hat to be put on or taken off when it makes other people uncomfortable.

Your niece sounds like a perceptive and sensitive child. She must feel strongly about her decision to be a vegetarian despite her young age and lack of support at home. She must also admire you very much and consider you a role model whom she'd like to emulate. Outside influences, especially ones that contradict a parent's own perspective, can be aggravating and troublesome to deal with and explain. Nevertheless they are rampant, so parents are frequently compelled to contend with annoying issues even though they are irksome. Your veganism is only one obstacle among many that your sister will encounter as a parent.

Do not feel guilty about revealing who you are to your niece. It is your sister's responsibility to find a way to contend with her feelings about it and your niece's response to it, not yours. Your sister may be harboring feelings of remorse, shame, or confusion about eating meat, and your avoidance of meat in her presence may draw these emotions and her resentment about them to the surface. She may be miffed that her daughter doesn't eat the food she prepares, and she may be at a loss regarding what to cook for her instead. Disclosing your veganism may further affect your niece's food choices, leaving your sister feeling more helpless and exasperated than before. In addition, if your niece believes that vegetarianism is right and eating meat is wrong, your sister might wonder how this will alter her daughter's opinion of her as a meat-eater.

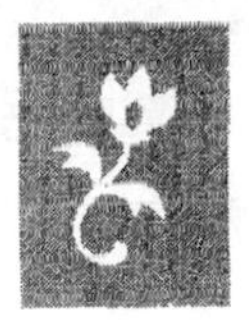

Veganism is the sum of a person's character. It is not a hat to be put on or taken off when it makes other people uncomfortable.

You can tell your sister that you simply cannot comply with her desire for you to hide your vegan ethics. Explain that it would feel like lying and that you always want to be honest and open with your niece. Then ask her why this is so problematic for her. It is important that the two of you have a candid dialogue about this matter so you can clear the air of hostility and buried anger. Try to find out the true source of her anxiety–fear, embarrassment, lack of information, concern for her daughter's health, or something else. Try to be empathic without compromising who you are and how you feel about being vegan. Explore ways that you could be of assistance to your sister should your niece decide to become vegan in the future, and ask how you might be of help to her now that her daughter has already chosen to be vegetarian.

Remember that your niece is exposed to many ideas from a multitude of sources. She has a mind of her own, and you may not be the only impetus for her decision to be vegetarian or vegan. In addition, your sister's frustrations may stem from more than this single issue.

Regardless of her reticence, she needs to see that her daughter's determination to demonstrate compassion ought to be a point of pride, not pain. Your own joy and exuberance about being vegan could inspire your sister to look beyond the hassles of having a vegan or vegetarian daughter and to consider the rewards and satisfaction of parenting a child with a conscience and a heart.

This has happened to me several times and it frustrates me to no end. I was talking to my mother about how important my beliefs regarding veganism are to me, and every time I'd say something to explain how I feel, she'd diminish it by saying, "Well, what about the atrocities done to humans? If I were going to spend any of my time on a cause, I'd focus on people issues first. After all, people are much more important than animals."

My parents think that just because I've chosen to focus my pursuits toward animal compassion, I'm choosing nonhuman animals over humans. I tell them that I am not choosing. I am against inflicting pain and suffering on any being, be it animal or human. I am only one person, though, and I can't fix all the world's problems by myself. The issue that tends to take the forefront on my personal agenda is veganism because it affects so many aspects of life. How can I deal with people who contend that vegans should spend their time on more direct human problems?

What you describe is an interesting scenario that some omnivores pose when they want to deflect attention away from their own habits and transfer any guilt they may harbor about them onto the vegan. It is illogical to think that since we can't spend all our time helping other people, we should continue to abuse and slaughter animals. There is absolutely no correlation between the two issues. A person can be vegan *and* help people. Compassion, according to vegan principles, accords no hierarchy of lesser or greater value to any living being. To vegans, all life is equally precious.

It is easy to advance rote theories such as "humans are more important than animals" when they are to our benefit. Nevertheless, there is nothing to support such conjecture. Worth is in the eye of the beholder.

Compassion, according to vegan principles, accords no hierarchy of lesser or greater value to any living being. To vegans, all life is equally precious.

People create and amend their perspectives relative to what they want and what they think will give them the greatest advantage in the world. Unfortunately, such rationalizations have led to some of the worst human atrocities, including slavery, war, ethnic cleansing, and the persecution, slaughter, and decimation of countless other species.

Essentially all the problems facing both humans and animals today have been created by people. In addressing these concerns, vegans choose to help the most needy and defenseless, those who have no resources to counter our assaults.

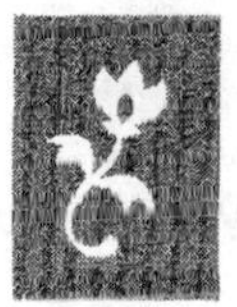

It is illogical to think that since we can't spend all our time helping other people, we should continue to abuse and slaughter animals.

No matter what any of us would do to help people *or* animals, it would never be quite enough because as individuals we are simply incapable of addressing all the rampant injustices that exist in the world. Consequently, we each must use our time and energies wisely and in ways that correspond with our convictions.

It is unfair for anyone to judge what another sees as her or his life's calling and purpose. When these kinds of comments are hurled in your direction, try to bear in mind the motivation behind them. There is no point in debating nonsensical remarks that spring from an irrational premise. Do your best to ignore them, because there is no effective way to counter them with reason.

Recently, at twenty-three, I have come to the decision that a total vegetarian diet is the right choice for me. I have moved in with my sister, her husband, and their soon-expected child. How do I deal with cooking meat dinners for them when it is against my own beliefs?

Unless this topic was discussed previously with your family, your decision to become a vegetarian will most likely startle or perplex them. Also, they might be angry if, as part of your living arrangement, you had agreed to prepare meals for everyone. However, since you have come to certain revelations of conscience, you should follow your heart and not compromise your newfound beliefs.

The only way to deal with this dilemma is to be honest and direct with your sister and brother-in-law. Let them know as soon as possible about your decision to be a vegetarian, and explain that you would find cooking meat unbearable. If you feel strongly about your convictions, you may be unwilling to bend on this point. Nevertheless, there may be other options that the three of you could explore. Here are a few ideas:

- Your sister or her husband could prepare a meat dish for themselves the prior evening or in the morning and you could just put it in the oven for them at dinnertime.
- They could cook a few meat dishes on the weekend and eat them throughout the week along with whatever vegetarian dishes you would prepare.
- You could cook vegetarian dinners during the week and they could prepare meat-based meals for themselves on the weekend.
- While you are fixing vegetarian selections, they could make a separate meat dish.
- They could purchase prepared meats or meat-based entrées and supplement them with your vegetarian dishes.

If you brainstorm together, you will be able to think of additional possibilities that would fit everyone's schedule and needs. Of course, there is always a chance that your family will be excited about meals that seem more healthful to them, especially in light of your sister's pregnancy. They may be delighted that you are eager and able to provide nutritious vegetarian alternatives.

Approach your sister and her husband with love and concern, without apologizing for your choices. Be open to their suggestions and be willing to offer your own. As long as everyone has one another's best interests at heart, a workable plan will be achieved.

I am a vegan who just got engaged to a vegan. We are planning our wedding and my first inclination was to make it a vegan one. My future mother-in-law said that for a lot of people a vegan meal might not be enjoyable, and do I really want to impose my beliefs on others? I realize that this wedding is for the families as well as my fiancée and myself, and that they and many others would be happier with an alternative, but I am not comfortable with serving meat and dairy. What should I do?

For many people, weddings are a major social event and an opportunity to publicly pull out all the stops to celebrate with friends and relatives. One of the reasons nonvegan parents often balk at the idea of a vegan wedding is the fear of embarrassment. They may believe that vegan food is bland, unappetizing, or unsatisfying. They may be concerned about looking like tightwads, since animal-based foods are still cultural symbols of affluence. They may feel they'll have to apologize to their guests for not serving meat. They may also be troubled that people will talk behind their backs after the wedding.

For the vast majority of people, eating meat is a personal choice, not an ethical one and certainly not a physical necessity. Abstaining from eating animal products for a few hours will not present a moral conflict nor cause physical suffering for any of your guests. On the other hand, there is no ethical controversy posed by vegan foods. In other words, while you, your fiancee, and some of your guests may be morally outraged at the inclusion of animal products at your reception, no one would be offended by vegan fare and everyone can partake

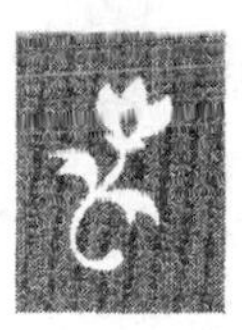

Eating meat is a personal choice, not an ethical one. On the other hand, there is no ethical controversy posed by vegan foods.

If your future mother-in-law is paying for the wedding and reception, she may feel that she has the right to make the final decision about what food is served. In this case, you and your fiancée could offer to pay for the reception or at least for the food at the reception. Instead of having a large wedding (if you were planning a large wedding), you could scale things down and invite only your closest friends and relatives, who would more readily be aware of your vegan lifestyle and would expect a vegan reception. Another idea is to have a vegan hors d'oeuvres reception with no meal following. Many popular and elegant hors d'oeuvres are naturally vegan, and there are many imaginative possibilities. Here are just a few ideas: teriyaki vegetables in vegan crepes, marinated artichoke hearts in filo packets, bite-size vegan egg rolls with a mustard or sweet-sour sauce, stuffed or fried exotic mushrooms, vegan spanokopita, mini vegetable kebobs, crostini, hummus and baba ganoush with pita triangles, nut pâté, vegan pesto, roasted vegetables, guacamole, breaded zucchini strips, vegetable tempura, polenta squares with fresh fruit salsa, potato pancakes with fresh herbs, rice- and pignolia-stuffed grape leaves, or angel hair pasta with spicy peanut sauce. The possibilities are unlimited.

If your future mother-in-law is mostly concerned that vegan entrées won't look appealing or taste good, and these are the only issues holding her back from consenting to a vegan meal, you could consult with local caterers (bring recipes, if necessary) to see what they might be able to whip up. Many creative chefs relish the chance to do something out of the ordinary, and some areas even have caterers who specialize solely in vegan cuisine. They may be able to provide a formal tasting of a few alternatives, which would let everyone evaluate their presentation skills as well as try the food. Providing menu suggestions and food samplings may allay any fears about vegan food not being delicious or satisfying. This in itself is often enough to transform a skeptic's point of view.

These, of course, are not your only options. Together, you, your fiancée, and her mother may be able to brainstorm even more possibilities that would allow everyone to feel comfortable. When you work together, taking into account the interests and feelings of the others involved, you will be doing more than just resolving your current dilemma. You will be establishing a compassionate standard for future communications that will make your relationship more respectful and honest–bringing to life the true spirit of veganism.

I am in my mid-twenties and don't live at home. I am finishing graduate school next month, and my mother wants to throw a party for me. While she intends on providing a few vegan entrées and desserts for me, she thinks it is totally unfair to expect others to eat vegan. I don't want to appear ungrateful, but since it is a party in my honor, I would feel most honored if a vegan meal were served. Should I grit my teeth and lighten up? If not, are there any suggestions for dealing with this sensitively?

It is very generous of your mother to want to celebrate your graduation with a party. Whether or not you should insist on it being vegan depends on how strongly you feel. Many people who are unfamiliar with vegan food are frightened that it would be sparse and dull when they would much prefer something festive and elegant. They usually don't realize that vegan fare can be just as sumptuous as food that contains animal products, if not more so. If there are enough options available, and the food is presented well and tastes good, few omnivores will even notice that the menu is animal-free.

Talk to your mom about your preferences. Work up a tentative menu or discuss your situation with a vegan caterer. Then submit your suggestions to her and offer to prepare or arrange for a tasting so she can see and sample some of the possibilities. Frequently, high-quality food is all it takes to win someone over to the idea of an all-vegan affair.

One meatless meal one day out of the year isn't too much to ask a meat-eater to endure, and your guests might just discover some scrumptious new dishes they'd like to have again. If you and your mother don't mention that the food is vegan, no one will be the wiser. As long as everything is attractive, tasty, and filling, the guests will be happy.

If you would be miserable with nonvegan food at a party intended to laud your accomplishments, then don't compromise who you are. If your mother is unwilling to spring for an all-vegan party, tell her "thanks, but no thanks." Let her know that you greatly appreciate her loving and thoughtful gesture, but you would be deeply disturbed and saddened if meat or other animal products were purchased and served in your "honor."

Vegan Etiquette

My family and I recently moved to a new town, into a neighborhood known for its friendliness. However, we weren't prepared to handle a local welcoming committee that came bearing gifts of food (mostly meat and dairy dishes) soon after we arrived. Of course they had no way of knowing that we are vegans. How could we turn down their generous offering? We didn't want to seem ungrateful or hurt anyone's feelings, especially when first meeting. So, we accepted, said thank you, and then discreetly gave the food to a nonvegan acquaintance. Consequently, we were the ones that ended up feeling bad. How can we explain to these neighbors now that we never eat animal products?

It's invariably difficult to handle surprise situations with aplomb. Nevertheless, honest communication from the outset can quash many potential problems. Had you been candid with your neighbors initially, you could have averted this unpleasant and somewhat embarrassing circumstance.

In retrospect, it's always much easier to think of what we might have done differently. You and your family maneuvered a disturbing predicament with sensitivity to your neighbors' warm welcome. Now, however, you are faced with the aftermath of managing future interactions.

If you don't anticipate regular or significant contact with your neighbors, it may not be necessary to tell them you are vegan. But if you intend to have any kind of relationship with them, this defensive tactic will only prolong the inevitable. To thrive, friendship requires tact and truth. Therefore, it is imperative that you and your family are frank about your diet and lifestyle.

The simplest and most direct approach is to talk to each neighbor individually. Speak openly and straightforwardly from your heart. Let them know that you were caught off guard and were confused about how to handle the situation. Apologize up front for not being forthright, and voice your thanks for their thoughtfulness and generosity.

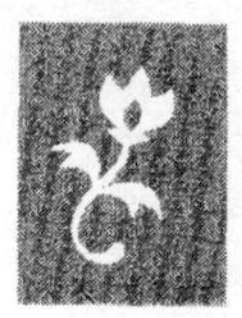

To thrive, friendship requires tact and truth. Honest communication from the outset can quash many potential problems.

You may be asked about what happened to the food. Fortunately, giving it to a meat-eating acquaintance is a perfectly reasonable explanation. (No one wants to hear that their heirloom recipe became the dog's lunch or was composted into garden mulch!)

There is no painless solution to this dilemma. To set things right, you must swallow your pride and take the initiative. Your honesty in expressing your own sense of awkwardness combined with your deep appreciation for their reception should make for a positive induction into this caring community.

I recently spent a weekend with an old fraternity buddy that I'd been out of touch with for twenty years. Since I knew that we'd be sharing some meals, I called him prior to the visit to tell him that I had become a vegan and explained in great detail what I do and do not eat. I let him know that I didn't want him or his wife to go to a lot of trouble to accommodate my food and suggested some easy options. All was going well until the first meal—dinner. The entrée was clearly a vegetable and pasta dish, but what about that dark gravy topping and the creamy-looking soup? I learned upon questioning that the gravy was made with beef bouillon and the soup was canned cream of mushroom with dairy ingredients. They obviously still didn't understand my diet. I told them it was no big deal and ended up eating the salad with some vegan crackers. My friend was apologetic and seemed okay with things. However, his wife seemed cooler during the rest of the weekend. Is there anything I could have done to avoid this unfortunate situation?

First of all, you're assuming something went wrong and that you were the cause of it. Without asking your friend's wife directly about your concern, there is no way to know for certain what, if anything, was bothering her. Sometimes moods are easily misinterpreted, especially with people we don't know very well. There are many possible causes for someone's change in demeanor. For instance, a headache, stress, illness, a disturbing phone call, or a spat with one's spouse or family could try the temperament of even the most good-natured person.

For people unacquainted with vegan living, sorting out what's appropriate to serve can be overwhelming. If you are the only vegan your friends know, their incentive to understand vegan dietary needs is likely limited. Next time you plan a sojourn with nonvegetarian friends, bring along a few nonperishable food items just in case. If time permits, send ahead a few simple recipes prior to your visit. You could also pack your favorite cookbook or recipes and offer to prepare a meal or two for everyone during your stay.

Occasionally, we all encounter people who are intimidated by vegans and vegetarians, often for a multitude of reasons. On some level, they may be aware of their own inhumane or unhealthful eating habits. Knowing that you have successfully adopted a more peaceful and health-supporting way of life can seem threatening. Furthermore, they may think that their kitchen and cooking skills are being scrutinized. They may regard themselves as ignorant and unknowledgeable about vegetarianism, especially when they are around you. Complicating matters further, they might be embarrassed or feel guilty about their own dietary choices, and may direct anger toward the person they deem responsible for making them feel this way—you.

If you are planning to maintain ongoing contact with your old friend and his wife, it may be worthwhile for your own peace of mind and your friendship to find out if you inadvertently perturbed her. The best approach is the direct one: Call her. After conveying your gratitude for their hospitality, ask her gently but candidly if you did anything that might have upset her. Tactfully tell her that you sensed a bit of distance after dinner your first night together, and you were concerned that you might have been the cause. Maintain an open, friendly, nonaccusatory tone, keeping in mind that you might have simply misread things. Regardless of the explanation, let her save face. Accept any apology she offers with understanding and grace, or offer your own if circumstances warrant, even though you may feel you did nothing wrong.

If you do not intend to continue the relationship or if you expect your contact to be minimal, send a thank-you note or small gift to acknowledge their kindness during your visit. Express your appreciation sincerely. Then, shine a light on your higher wisdom and let the incident go.

What is a polite way to tell a host my dietary preferences upon accepting a dinner invitation?

It is always thoughtful and courteous to tell the host your dietary constraints as soon as possible after an invitation has been extended. Few things are as disconcerting at a dinner party (for both the guest and the host) than for a guest to find nothing suitable to eat.

There's no shortcut to disclosing the fact that you're vegan. Be honest but tactful in your approach. Explain briefly what being vegan means in terms of your diet. Let your host know what specific items are and are not acceptable. Remember, this may be the host's first encounter with such an "unconventional" way of eating, so she or he may be puzzled as to what to prepare for you.

Reach out to your host as much as possible. Mention some commonplace vegan foods the host might want to prepare. Offer to supply some simple vegan recipes for the event–as an adjunct to the non-vegan foods that will be served, not as a replacement–or suggest preparing a dish to bring with you when you come. Some hosts are offended by guests bringing a dish to their event, feeling that this could imply they are incompetent. Try to be sensitive to this issue and do what you can to find a comfortable solution for both you and your host.

Most hosts are anxious to be as accommodating as possible once they clearly understand what to buy or fix for a vegan. If your host doesn't want to cook something special and seems uneasy with the idea of you making a supplemental dish, recommend a few brand-name vegan products or locally prepared vegan foods and let the host know which nearby stores carry them.

If, even after speaking with the host, you are concerned you'll leave the party hungry, eat a light meal before you go. Don't fill up too much, though. In case your host pleasantly surprises you with lots of vegan goodies, you'll want to be sure you still have plenty of appetite left to show your enthusiastic appreciation.

I was recently invited to a wedding where I know there will be no vegan food. The ceremony is scheduled for the late afternoon and the reception and sit-down dinner will go well into the night. I am concerned about being hungry for such a long time, so I'm thinking about packing some food in my purse to eat in the ladies' room. Does this sound like a reasonable solution or is there something else I could do?

A wedding is a milestone for the bride and groom, but it is also a celebration with family and friends. Most couples want their guests to have a fun time and enjoy themselves. In addition to being the highlight of the party, the newlyweds are also the hosts, so it is important to them that their guests are comfortable and don't go hungry.

Wedding plans usually involve attending to numerous details and coordinating endless tasks. With sufficient notice, however, one more special request won't ruin the occasion or detract from their day. After all, the couple is paying for your meal anyway, and they surely don't want to see it go to waste. Caterers are often very creative and don't mind accommodating a vegan guest. On the other hand, eating in the lavatory would be unseemly.

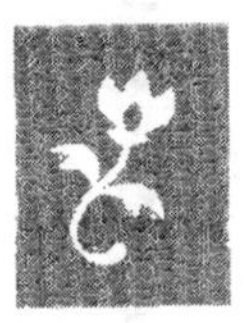

Being vegan is nothing to be ashamed about,
and there is no need to apologize for your beliefs.

Talk to the couple frankly and explain your dietary needs. If they are friends or family members, they will understand. Being vegan is nothing to be ashamed or embarrassed about, and you don't need to apologize for your beliefs. They probably will be very happy that you trusted them enough to confide in them, and you will be relieved to know that a suitable meal will be prepared without a hassle. But don't wait until the last minute. Try to give the bride and groom as much notice as possible. This way they will have time to make the arrangements without creating extra stress for themselves or frazzling the caterer. Despite any trepidation you may have, your honesty and consideration will be appreciated.

I work in a large office and, as far as I know, am the only vegan. Any tips for dealing with group lunches, either in a restaurant or in a conference room?

If you've worked in the office for any length of time, chances are your coworkers have already observed your uncommon eating habits, so learning that you are vegan will probably come as no surprise. A broad disclosure, however, could lead to undesirable comments, teasing, or just a slew of questions, all of which can be distracting and annoying. In addition, broadcasting personal information in the workplace is usually interpreted as inappropriate and unprofessional.

If you are comfortable talking to the individual who selects the restaurants or orders food for your business meetings, speak with that person privately and discuss your concerns. It actually may be quite easy to choose alternatives that will provide acceptable options for everyone without singling you out unnecessarily. She or he might even request your input about what foods to serve at meetings or which restaurants are vegan friendly. You could mention that there are probably a number of other employees who also would be grateful for animal-free alternatives, including people who are simply concerned about eating more healthfully.

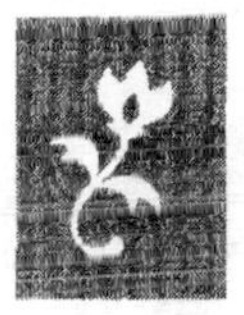

The office is not a smart place to preach "the vegan gospel."

If you are friendly with some of the other workers who attend these luncheon gatherings, let them know how much you would appreciate their support. Suggest they join you occasionally in ordering vegan items so you don't feel like the odd one out. If you've been vegan for a while, you know how omnivores typically ogle our vegetable plates, pasta dishes, and salads, often dropping comments like, "Ooooh, that looks delicious. I should have ordered what you're having." So, it may not be all that difficult to convince a few others to come on board, even if it's only for an intermittent meal or snack.

Some business situations may require you to frequent restaurants without being forewarned or without being given a choice of establishments, and you could be put in a tight spot. Call ahead, if possible, to find out if any vegan options are already on the menu or if the chef could prepare a standard dish without the nonvegan ingredients or could whip up an expressly vegan creation. Bear in mind that some chefs are overwhelmed by having to make an out-of-the-ordinary concoction, particularly at busy lunch or dinner times. On the other hand, many chefs rise to the occasion and relish the chance to be inventive. When you are unable to call ahead, try to speak with your server discreetly so as not to attract attention. Ideally, sit among colleagues who know you are vegan so you can discuss your needs with the waitstaff more openly.

When worse comes to worst, you can always order a vegetable salad. If there is concern about your co-workers raising their eyebrows, try to keep your choice low key. It's not necessary to make a fuss. Even if you're obliged to visit a steak house, you can generally get a good salad bowl and plain baked potato. However, salads and other light meals may not be very satisfying when you're particularly hungry, so keep a quick snack in your briefcase or desk drawer for such emergencies.

Sometimes even the best intentions fall flat; for instance, the day the whole gang decides to order in cheese pizza without your knowledge. It's a good idea to keep some nonperishable snacks and heat-and-eat meals on hand to have *before* a lunch meeting if there's any concern that nothing would be available for you to eat. This way you won't be ravenous going into an unpredictable situation.

The office is not a smart place to preach "the vegan gospel," so be selective in what you say, how you say it, and to whom. Proselytizing is often tempting but rarely welcome. With just a little creativity, it's possible to be respectful of your colleagues and the corporate milieu while honoring and maintaining your vegan beliefs.

I watch some kids on the weekends at their house, but I haven't told their mother that I'm vegan. It goes against my beliefs to feed them all the garbage they eat. Any thoughts as to what I can do?

There are two issues at hand here: your own personal beliefs and your objection to preparing and serving animal-based foods for the children you watch. You are entitled to follow your ethics and practice veganism because it is a private choice that you are not thrusting on anyone outside yourself. A problem arises, however, when an individual's personal convictions are imposed on others.

The best time to have discussed this with the mother was before you accepted the position since it appears that one of the requirements is to feed the children what she wants them to have. Aside from your feelings about the job, it is important that you make some pivotal decisions:

- Are you willing to remain in your present capacity if you are obliged to serve animal products to the children?
- If the mother consents to you giving the children vegan options, how would you respond if they won't eat the foods you offer, or if they tell you they want meat and dairy products?
- Are you willing and financially able to resign from your post if the situation doesn't change?

People should not be forced to prepare foods that are disturbing for them to handle. Conversely, childcare workers are constrained to feed their charges what their parents request. Discuss your concerns with the children's mother. She might be more receptive to the idea of vegan meals for the kids than you anticipate. On the other hand, she could remain adamant that you feed them the meat-based diet to which they are accustomed. In this case, if you feel unable to acquiesce to the mother's wishes, you might be better off looking for a different position.

Friends and Strangers

I am a senior in high school. I'm finding it harder and harder to be around meat-eaters who have no concern for the animals they consume. How do I deal with friends who refuse to stop bugging me about my diet, lifestyle, and compassion for all animals?

Because at times it can be painful to be around meat-eaters, some vegans prefer to keep company only with other vegans. Although this is understandable, it minimizes options and closes off relationships that could otherwise bring joy to our lives. Our nonvegan pals have many positive attributes that caused us to seek them out as friends in the first place. These qualities do not change simply because our own view of the world has shifted. Our friends have remained the same—we are the ones who have moved in a different direction.

Instead of being frustrated that your buddies have not chosen the same path you have, you can help them understand your point of view by calmly sharing with them your reasons for being vegan. They will be able to hear what you are saying and think about the issues more objectively if they do not feel put down, pressured, or attacked in the process. Your friends will most likely be more tolerant of your choice if you demonstrate the same nonjudgmental consideration toward them that you hope to receive. If, despite your efforts, their taunting persists and you find it too distressing to bear, let them know in a composed, rational tone how it makes you feel. They may be completely oblivious to how much their comments hurt you. If the derision continues in spite of your explanation, you may need to sacrifice their friendship, at least for the time being, and start to develop relationships with people who are more open-minded and accepting of you.

I am often faced with responding to people's questions about my lifestyle and was wondering if you have a few short but sweet responses that work and get to the point. I find that people often get defensive, which is not my goal. But I get frustrated because I just don't think people understand where I am coming from.

The scenario you describe is one that most vegans encounter sooner or later, but there is no single best way to handle it. Nonvegans generally ask questions about veganism for one of two reasons: genuine curiosity, or as a way to justify their own chosen diet or lifestyle. When people inquire about veganism because they sincerely desire to learn something about it, they rarely become defensive. However, when people are disparaging in the course of their investigation, it's a clue that they are more interested in devaluing veganism as a means to vindicate conventional thought. Usually it's not meant as a personal attack, even though it inevitably feels that way.

Responses can be short and to the point, humorous, or vague. The choice really hinges on your style and how you are most comfortable communicating. Your reply should also depend on whether or not the individual asking the questions is actually engrossed in your answers or just harassing you. Remember that you do not owe anyone an explanation, and you do not have to defend your way of life.

The most effective rejoinders are usually those that are brief and upbeat. Here is one possibility: "I believe in the value of all life and in not harming others. Since we can live healthfully and happily without eating or using animal products, there is no reason to do otherwise." Usually this is enough to satisfy those who do not really want to know more, and it allows them to retain their dignity in the process.

Vegans frequently feel they are obligated to delve into the details of their lifestyle and philosophy as a means of educating others. Although this may be enlightening, unless someone is personally motivated to hear about alternative ways of living and is also willing to maintain an open heart and mind, your words will be just so much hot air. The conversation will then turn into a painful test of your tolerance, patience, and self-control.

It's useless to try to get people to grasp your point of view if they are overly protective of their own. In these cases, offer a short but pleasant comment, and then move away from the topic as quickly and gracefully as possible. If they truly want to explore it further, they'll let you know.

Where can vegans meet other vegans?

Vegans can be found in almost all areas of North America and in many parts of the world, even remote or oppressive places where it might seem impossible to be vegan. But because the only attribute that differentiates vegans from anyone else is the application of our ethic, vegans are often anonymous, even to each other.

As with any cultural minority, it is easier to sustain one's beliefs and lifestyle when supported by others who share the same convictions. National vegan, vegetarian, and animal rights organizations do an excellent job of creating a sense of unity and camaraderie despite their affiliates being scattered in many directions. Some groups produce periodicals, such as newsletters or magazines, and include a free subscription with each membership. This can provide not only enjoyable reading matter and insightful articles, but also access to information about local and national conferences, events, and other gatherings where vegans come together. Some publications contain a listing of regional contacts, people who have volunteered to be resource points for local or visiting vegans.

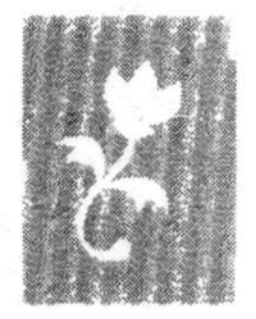

As with any cultural minority, it is easier to sustain one's beliefs and lifestyle when supported by others who share the same convictions.

In large and midsize cities there are usually several natural food stores and food cooperatives. Occasionally these establishments sponsor workshops, lectures, or social events that can range from informative to all-out festive. Generally a large proportion of vegetarians and vegans comprise the audience. Many of these stores also have bulletin boards and newsletters that provide listings of local activist groups, vegan and vegetarian get-togethers and share-a-dish meals, meetings of the local chapters of national vegetarian and animal rights organizations, vegetarian societies, and so forth. These notices can alert you to what is happening in your area and put you in touch with like-minded people.

For those who live in small towns and rural areas, it is much harder to find other vegans. Frequently, hamlets and villages are situated in or near "food animal" farms and hunting areas where the prospect of veganism is typically met with hostility. In this case, it may be necessary to travel occasionally to the nearest large town or city that has a natural food store to find out what groups and activities, if any, are available there for vegans. Of course, people can always try to start their own group or establish a local chapter of a national organization, but in outlying areas this is usually quite a challenge.

The Internet can be a terrific way to connect with other vegans, and you might meet others who live fairly close to you. Even if you don't develop real-time friendships through this medium, cyber-pals can commiserate with your situation and offer a great deal of support and understanding. Vegan discussion boards and mailing lists are helpful for maintaining awareness of other perspectives. They also can involve vegans in stimulating on-line dialogues. Web sites provide access to endless information and can help notify vegans about upcoming events and activities.

Part of seeking out other vegans means taking the initiative. Use every opportunity you have to investigate who and what is available to you and be an active participant. If you make the effort to reach out to other vegans, you'll find many wonderful people just waiting to reach back.

My best friend invited my family to a traditional Thanksgiving celebration. I turned her down, and she came back a few days later offering to have a vegan feast instead. When her old friends were told of the change in menu, they reacted with extreme hostility, and now the whole thing is off. I want so much to do something to help my friend deal with her friends' animosity, but I feel lost. Any suggestions?

Many people are indoctrinated with nostalgic sentiment about the holidays, so it was bold and thoughtful of your friend to offer to prepare a vegan Thanksgiving. Your friendship must be very important to her, and she obviously respects your convictions, even though she doesn't share them.

When the family or friends of a vegan are adamant about having a meat-centered celebration in spite of the vegan's protestations, they often are making several unspoken assertions:

1. They presume that meat-eaters should not be made to feel uncomfortable and therefore should not be forced to sacrifice their dietary indulgences.
2. They believe that meat is central to the celebration and that it wouldn't be any fun without it.
3. If they are willing to sacrifice the vegan's attendance because they want to maintain the turkey tradition, they are in essence

stating that the food or other guests take precedence over the vegan's company.

4. They surmise that a vegan feast wouldn't be appealing, exciting, or satisfy their appetite.

Most vegans are deeply upset by the sight of a dead animal at the hub of a supposed festive occasion. For activists who work all year long to educate others about the horrors of the slaughter industries, this can be especially distressing. In a culture where cadavers are prayed over and buried, not displayed and consumed, a vegan is more likely to grieve than rejoice.

Oftentimes meat-eaters believe that vegans should be satisfied as long as they have something to eat. They are unaware that for most vegans, watching others gnaw on body parts causes anguish and revulsion. On the other hand, a vegan feast offends no one. Everyone can partake because there is nothing immoral about not serving products of death. In addition, when the guests all share the same food, instead of the vegan being served something different, it adds to a sense of conviviality and camaraderie.

If the group had a history of spending Thanksgiving together, they may have felt that a vegan event would spoil their established custom. They may have thought your friend was showing favoritism and were offended that perhaps she prefers you over them. Also, the way your friend informed the other people may have influenced their reaction. Many meat-eaters know very little about veganism and have their own preconceived notions that vegans subsist on lettuce and carrot sticks–not very appetizing fare for a feast. They may have been indignant, thinking that a vegan repast would leave them feeling hungry and deprived.

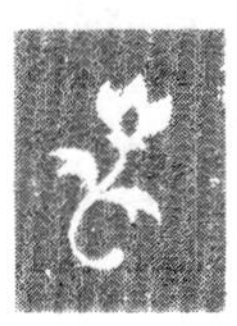

Oftentimes meat-eaters believe that vegans should be satisfied as long as they have something to eat. They are unaware that for most vegans, watching others gnaw on body parts causes anguish and revulsion.

Even though you were the catalyst for the change in venue and feel lousy about the aftermath, you are not responsible for your best friend's feelings or for the callous treatment she received from her other friends. True friendship does not dissolve the instant something goes awry. People who care about each other talk things out, try to understand the other's point of view, and give as well as take. Her fair-weather pals failed miserably when their friendship was put to the test. Even if they felt that you were being given preferential treatment or that your friend favored you over them, it does not excuse their immature and insensitive behavior.

Your friend made a choice to support you and defend your beliefs. There was no guarantee that the group would be receptive. She took a risk on your behalf, but that does not make you culpable. You can demonstrate your gratitude by comforting your friend and offering solace and a sympathetic ear. However, you cannot erase the heartache she feels over her friends' rancor. It is unfortunate that you are bearing the brunt of this sad situation, but the discord is between her and her other friends. They are the ones who must be held accountable for the dissolution or recovery of their relationship, not you.

I am trying to get the people around me to understand why I am vegan, but I am not doing a very good job. They are constantly harassing me about it at every meal, and I am tired of it. I want them to stop, but I don't know how to approach them without being rude. What should I do?

Most teasing by friends and family is not provoked by malice. Nevertheless, the distress it can cause is very real. There are typically three reasons why people tease. In many instances, the underlying aim of good-natured needling is to strengthen the bond of friendship. Inside jokes can draw friends closer because they are sharing privileged information. Occasionally the catalyst is a need to vent some steam. Humor can force friends to let down their guard and shake off any anxiety about their differences. Quips that are designed to rankle, however, are rarely amusing.

When teasing turns to taunting it is usually spurred by scorn. Yet below the surface is often a layer of fear, ignorance, insecurity, or shame. Many people are aware of veganism to one degree or another, and with growing media exposure it is becoming more difficult to conceal the horrors of the slaughter industries. On a certain level, friends and family who harass you about your vegan beliefs may be expressing misgivings about their own dietary choices. You are a constant cue that they eat animals—a point that the majority of omnivores would rather ignore. Whether their concerns are for personal health or virtue, your presence reminds them of issues they would prefer to relegate to the depths of their subconscious.

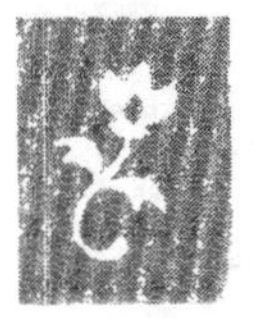

Most teasing by friends and family is not provoked by malice. Nevertheless, the distress it can cause is very real.

Frequently people do not realize that their comments are offensive. One way to handle it is to ask them point-blank to stop. Let them know that you don't appreciate their remarks because being vegan is a serious matter to you.

If the kidding appears to be out of genuine caring, not rancor, another approach is to lighten up and laugh along with the group. Sometimes joining the banter is enough to prompt it to end. When others see that their razzing no longer bothers you, it will either deflate their fun and they'll turn their attention elsewhere, or they'll feel a stronger connection with you from having joined together in laughter. For those who are truly acting out of contempt, there is little you can do to turn them around. The most prudent way to protect yourself is to ignore them.

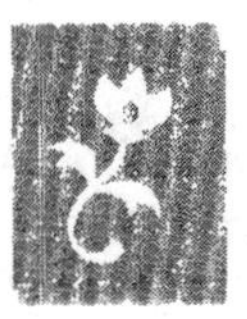

Verbally beating people into submission will not force open their ears or heart.

Virtually all vegans want those close to them to understand their commitment and motivation. But to people who aren't interested, preaching just makes them ill at ease and causes them to cease listening. If your friends and family demonstrate a genuine interest in your veganism, then you have a golden opportunity to educate. However, verbally beating people into submission will not force open their ears or heart. If there is no real curiosity, you are only wasting your energy and emotions.

People often get offended when I tell them that I am a vegan. They think that I do it just to be a nuisance or because it's the popular thing to do. How can I make them understand that being vegan is what is best for the animals, the planet, and our species?

Knowledge can affect people only if their minds and hearts are open to it. Those who are disinterested will not be influenced regardless of the zeal of the messenger. It can take an enormous amount of emotional energy to try to convince an apathetic person that what you have to say is important when she or he couldn't care less. Most longtime vegans come to realize this and tailor their efforts accordingly by focusing on attentive audiences that express sincere curiosity.

It is not necessary that others understand your beliefs for you to feel comfortable around them. However, it is vital that they respect you by not ridiculing your choices or asking you to defend them. Generally, people who deride vegans are uninformed, embarrassed about their own lifestyle, in a state of denial, or feeling threatened. People who are secure in themselves are more likely to ask questions out of a genuine desire to learn and will also be more open to hearing you talk about your reasons for becoming vegan. I created a "veganism" (a compassionate version of a conventional maxim) that addresses these types of predicaments. It goes as follows: Don't sing your song to a stone.

Sometimes the best way to handle a situation is to disregard it. Try not to draw attention to yourself or make a big deal out of being vegan when you are in social settings. Be the finest example of kindness and compassion that you can muster, even in the face of hostility. Eventually, people will leave you alone, respect you, or see you as a curiosity. Then, when they inquire about your veganism, it will be because they are truly interested, not because it is forced on them. This will present the best opportunity for you to inform and educate gently, without preaching. In this way, the authentic seekers will become visible, and your song will be heard not by stones but by budding flowers.

Chapter 3

Ethical Practice

Coming to Our Senses

Veganism is about waking up, becoming aware, and climbing out of the fog that shields most people from animal suffering and death–horrors that are perpetuated solely for the sake of habit, comfort, and greed. For many vegans, this process is both exhilarating and disconcerting. As if rousing from a groggy sleep, vegans take notice of the wonder and beauty of the living world–its vibrance, resilience, and splendor–and see once again with the eyes of a child.

At the same time, this arousal is painful. Awareness is not limited to the appealing aspects of life; it also exposes the repugnant and hideous. Yet, seeing with eyes wide open fosters a clearer view of life's essence and promotes deep and purposeful inner growth. People who shield themselves from the raw side of reality never fully develop their tender and compassionate nature. Until the barbed edges of anguish cut through the superficial armor of the heart, empathy will remain a stranger.

When the heart is stirred, passions abound, so it is not surprising that many new vegans dive into this lifestyle with a vengeance. Once aware, what sane, caring person would not express fury over the rampant deception and chronic injustices that fuel our modern economies?

People who shield themselves from the raw side of reality never fully develop their tender and compassionate nature.

Immersed in exuberance, however, it is common for novice vegans to lose sight of the actual aim of veganism. A gentle awakening can lead to obsession if one forgets that compassion, not perfection, is the purpose of vegan living. Our world is not ideal. Consequently, a preoccupation with trying to attain the impossible is exhausting and can lead to disillusionment or abandonment of the vegan lifestyle.

As a crusade, ferreting out the tiniest remnants of animal products in our lives is pointless because in contemporary society it simply cannot be achieved. There are animal body parts, by-products, and derivatives in practically every commodity. If vegan attention is diverted to eliminating the last iota of animal products in our public and private cupboards, there will be no time or stamina left to focus on education and other activities that could be significantly more productive.

If it is not possible to totally divest our lives of animal products, then what is the purpose in only going partway? Is there any point to veganism at all?

Vegans are at the forefront of bringing forth a revolutionary perspective, one that the world is as yet unprepared to embrace. In all successful social movements, however, progressive ideas have initially been met with scorn. Denial and resistance are to be expected, possibly even invited, because they are necessary precursors to change. Achievement cannot always be measured by the accomplishment of a final objective; few activists actually survive to see all their goals materialized. Formulating concepts and setting strategies in motion are the genesis of cultural transition and an indispensable part of launching lasting transformation, even though the rewards may, on the surface, appear insignificant.

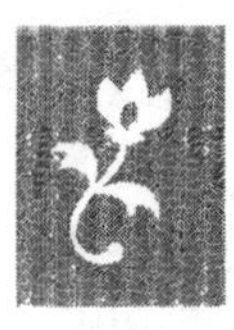

Vegans are at the forefront of bringing forth a revolutionary perspective, spurring a metamorphosis of spirit as well as substance.

Veganism is an all-encompassing ethic that infuses every aspect of a person's being. Unlike a mask, it cannot be removed whenever it becomes inconvenient or uncomfortable. For vegans, functioning in our nonvegan world can occasionally be awkward or perplexing, especially if circumstances don't present clear-cut vegan options. There are times when, try as we might, we must make concessions in order to manage effectively. Even when vegan theory and principles are patently understood, applying them is not always so simple.

This chapter explores a number of the large and small dilemmas that vegans commonly face and addresses some of the ethical predicaments we sometimes encounter. The questions tap into the sphere of compassion in which vegans find themselves. The answers provide possible pathways for consideration.

Advancing the Journey

I have been vegetarian for several years and would really love to go vegan. Apart from avoiding dairy products and other obviously animal-derived foods, what else do I need to do?

For most people, becoming vegan is a process, a series of steps and stages that continually bring the compassionate perspective into sharper focus. Longtime vegans rarely view their practice as a final destination. Rather, it is seen as an endless path, a stream of consciousness leading to deeper awareness.

Below is a code of vegan ethics that Stanley M. Sapon and I developed, which first appeared in *The Vegan Sourcebook.* It delineates the fundamental principles behind a vegan lifestyle and is followed by a few examples of how vegans put these ethics into daily practice.

A Code of Vegan Ethics

- *Vegans are sensitive to issues of suffering;* therefore, vegans shun actions that inflict pain on sensate, animate life, animal or human, either intentionally or thoughtlessly.
- *Vegans value the uniqueness of all life forms;* therefore, vegans seek to avoid wanton destruction of plant life and the exploitation of the physical environment in ways that endanger local or global ecosystems.
- *Vegans abjure violence;* therefore, vegans seek to deal with physical and social challenges in ways that are thoughtful, gentle, compassionate, considerate, and just.

- *Vegans expand the principle of harmlessness;* therefore, vegans strive for active beneficence, performing acts of kindness or charity.

Among the ways that vegans manifest their commitment to this code of ethics:

- Vegans choose foods that are exclusively plant-based.
- Vegans explicitly withhold economic and moral support from enterprises that exploit or abuse animals or humans.
- Vegans take care to choose those materials and products that neither destroy nor distort the lives of sensate creatures.
- Vegans actively reject the use of living creatures as instruments or materials for teaching, scientific inquiry, entertainment, or other utilitarian purposes.
- Vegans attempt to resolve conflict with sensitivity, respect, and nonviolent strategies.

To eventually become vegan, would one start out slowly, first as vegetarian, and then ease into veganism?

Approaches to veganism are as varied as vegans themselves. There is no best way to become vegan. It depends on your level of commitment and motivation as well as what you are most comfortable with. For many people, once they discover the realities behind their food and become aware of the widespread use of animal products in other areas of daily living, there is no choice but to make a rapid and complete conversion to veganism. Other people prefer a slower paced transition that allows them the opportunity to test the waters before diving in headfirst.

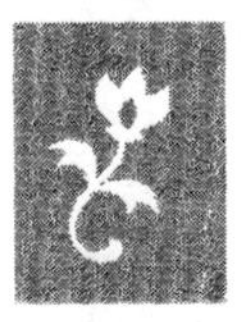

Veganism is a lifetime journey rather than an express destination.

When ethical vegetarians are confronted with the moral shortcomings of egg and dairy consumption, it is often enough to compel them to become vegan overnight. The production of eggs and milk entails as much cruelty, if not more so, as the production of flesh foods, because the animals' suffering is extended over a significantly longer period prior to their untimely and brutal slaughter. For many vegans, the barbarism involved in these industries makes the use of eggs and dairy products as repulsive as meat. Therefore, a vegetarian diet that includes these items is really not such a compassionate leap, as many people are led to believe.

Realistically speaking, most people go through a series of steps on the way to becoming vegan. Typically, diet is the first area of change and dairy products are often the final hurdle, after flesh foods and eggs. This process of elimination can take days, weeks, or months, depending on the individual's zeal. People who are vegetarians when they decide to become vegan may have a somewhat easier time than nonvegetarians, because they are already accustomed to alternative eating styles. However, this is not to suggest that it is necessary or even important to be a vegetarian before becoming vegan. It is simply a common pattern. What is right for someone else may not be right for you. Proceed at your own rate with a stride that corresponds to your degree of interest and personal determination. Once you make the decision to become vegan, your strategy will align with your incentive.

Vegan Limitations and Personal Choice

I've been wondering how to reconcile family heirlooms with the concept of veganism. I don't come from a wealthy family, and yet we have some precious items that I would feel terrible about discarding. As the only granddaughter, I received a pearl necklace from each of my grandmothers when I was in my teens. As they were passed to me, I hope to pass them on to future generations as treasured mementos of the women in our family. At present, I feel more uncomfortable about "unloading" the jewelry than I do about the murder of the mollusks. How can I square my ethical beliefs with the notion that I am being disrespectful to my family's matriarchs? Must I sell or give away the pearls to be considered vegan?

Many people inaccurately associate veganism with flawlessness when, in reality, it indicates a commitment to compassionate living and dynamic harmlessness, not perfection. There are no vegan police enforcing rigid laws of compassion and no vegan detectives snooping through our private possessions. Veganism resonates with kindness, caring, thoughtfulness, and respect for all life, including your own and the lives of your ancestors and descendants. The vegan ethic was not intended to cause harm or provoke suffering. If you are conflicted about parting with family heirlooms, something is out of kilter.

Try to step back from direct involvement with your dilemma to look at it objectively. How is your possession of the pearls causing harm? Would disposing of them make you feel worse than keeping them? How would selling them or giving them away demonstrate compassion? How can you bring balance to your predicament by respecting your family matriarchs while still honoring your vegan values?

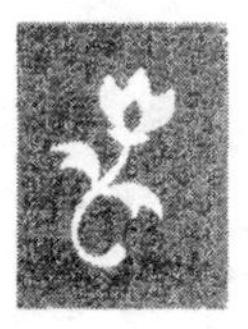

Veganism is a lifetime process that continually unfolds, ripens, and matures.

The pearls from your grandmothers carry deep sentimental worth for you. Holding on to them as a keepsake is not the same as buying new pearls or wearing them in public. One day you may decide to part with them, or you may choose to proceed with your present plan of passing them on to the next generation. If you do, you might want to accompany them with a tender explanation or perhaps a poem or other written words from you, so that the gift is made even more special and personalized and not focused specifically on the pearls.

Veganism is a lifetime journey without a sharp beginning or sudden end–the process continually unfolds, ripens, and matures. Each day vegans discover new ways to expand their humanity and extend their benevolence, but no one is expected to do everything all at once. Embrace your veganism moment by moment. Do not force changes on yourself; this will only make you resentful and sad. Acknowledge the transience of life and try to add meaning, purpose, joy, and compassion to all that you do. You already know the solution to your dilemma. Heed the quiet small voice inside you, for it is echoing your heart's desire.

I invited my friend to the movies, but he says he can't go because he is strictly vegan. He claims that the film itself contains animal products. I work in a movie theater and I know that the film is made of plastic. Could he perhaps be referring to the developing process? And would this same concern apply to photographic film?

Photographic film and movie film contain several layers of gelatin, which are an integral part of the film's chemistry. Gelatin is the protein derived from the bones, cartilage, tendons, skin, and other tissue of steer, calves, or pigs. Film is not the only communication medium that uses animal products. For instance, book glue is manufactured from collagenous materials made from animal hides or bones. Therefore the vast majority of books are not vegan.

In our present-day society, it is not really possible to a live a 100 percent pure vegan life—one that is totally harmless and includes no animal-derived products whatsoever—and still participate in the culture at large. It is sad that the use of animal products is so rampant. But because vegans comprise a small group with relatively limited power, we must assess where our efforts will have the most impact. If we work toward ending the source of materials for the by-products market—meat consumption—then we will be well on our way to abolishing our culture's reliance on animal-derived ingredients and materials.

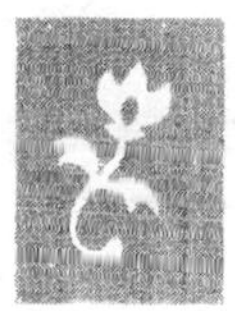

In our present-day society, it is not really possible to a live a 100 percent pure vegan life and still participate in the culture at large.

Certainly it is important to devise and use alternatives to animal-based commodities whenever possible. This said, we still need to evaluate what is currently available and use it to our advantage, if feasible. For example, books, photographs, and movies can be powerful documentary and educational tools that could positively influence individuals and groups and help redirect the course of our culture. Until there are suitable substitutes, we have no other options.

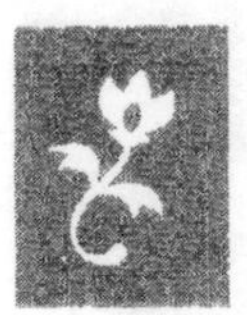

Being vegan is not about superiority or flawlessness, nor does it condemn practitioners to a spartan life of misery.

Being vegan is not about superiority or flawlessness, nor does it condemn practitioners to a spartan life of misery. For human beings to be whole and happy, we must have balance between our work and play, our joys and sorrows. Entertainment that does not involve exploitation can be valuable and is especially important for activists who are so often entrenched in the suffering of others. Going to the movies can be a pleasurable vegan activity (minus the buttered popcorn and milk chocolates, of course). Go grab your friend and enjoy!

As a vegan and an artist, I am very concerned about the materials I use for my artwork. I have tried to track down information on products used by oil painters such as paint, glue, oils, and mediums, but I have been unable to find out exactly where these items come from and how they are made.

Nearly all art supplies contain animal derivatives of one type or another. In addition, most formulations are proprietary and, since manufacturers of art supplies are not required to reveal their ingredients, very few do. It is understandable that you want to find cruelty-free products for your artwork, but, for now, it will most likely be a futile search. Even if you were to locate some products that were vegan, there is no guarantee they would be of the highest quality.

Using nonvegan art supplies is not necessarily a major problem that conflicts with vegan practice. We can only do what we are capable of and use those resources that are currently available. Manufacturers of art supplies are not directly exploiting animals. They use substances that are the by-products of the meat and dairy industries. These ingredients are cheap and have stood the test of time. Consequently, there is no incentive for manufacturers to seek out or devise alternatives.

Creative outlets are an essential part of a well-balanced life. Art is a glorious, expressive release for the artist, and artwork can bring joy, insight, and inspiration to vegans and nonvegans alike.

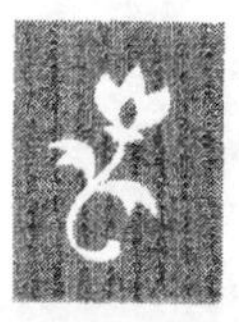

Creative outlets are an essential part of a well-balanced life and can help generate a more compassionate world.

Try not to get bogged down in the quest to eradicate every last speck of animal products from your life and look at the overall, long-term mission of veganism instead. As much as we may hope, a totally vegan world is not bound to evolve during our lifetime. Therefore, we must prioritize our efforts, use our potential wisely, and set reasonable objectives.

When we as a culture become more caring, art supplies will be made that are free of the residues of suffering and death. Use your energies to make changes that will have the greatest impact on generating a more compassionate world. Artwork, even if made with materials that contain some animal by-products, can be a valuable part of such a metamorphosis.

I am a vegan and have been a figure skater nearly all my life. About two years ago I bought a new pair of skates that are made fully of leather. I have been angry at myself ever since because of my selfishness in caring more about my personal enjoyment than an animal's life. I would love to continue my figure skating; it is a large part of my life. Over time, though, my feet have grown and my skates have broken down. To keep up my skating I must get new skates. The problem is that I need professional-quality, supportive boots. I have failed to find any supplier that produces vegan figure skates of this caliber. I have considered getting a pair custom made, but this would be extremely expensive. What should I do?

To make a decision you can live with, you need to weigh the options that are available to you. You could investigate getting synthetic leather custom boots to see if they are as expensive as you expect. Perhaps you will be pleasantly surprised to discover they are less costly than custom leather boots. If the cost is prohibitive and completely out of the range of your budget, then realistic vegan options are nonexistent.

It would be callous to suggest that you abandon your lifelong enjoyment of figure skating because you are unable to locate acceptable or affordable vegan skates. Taking care of yourself and ensuring that you have creative outlets that give you pleasure is not self-indulgent. In fact, this is vital for maintaining self-respect, self-esteem, and enjoyment of life, all important aspects of being wholly compassionate. If you are unable to find satisfactory vegan skates, then try to make the new leather ones that you purchase last as long as possible by repairing them and taking good care of them. Maybe by the time they are ready to be replaced, better alternatives will be available or you'll be more financially able to invest in a custom vegan pair.

Within many of the arts that vegans enjoy there are elements of lingering animal products for which no replacements have yet been devised. If we removed the expressive arts from vegans' lives, they would feel bleak and empty. Uplifting our heart and the hearts of those around us makes for a kinder and happier world. This is an important factor in vegan living, and no less significant than removing products of suffering from our lives.

By no means am I advocating buying a wardrobe of leather shoes. However, when essentially no feasible vegan options exist, buying one pair of leather skates may perhaps be less debilitating to your spirit than not skating at all.

Vegan Approaches to Hunger Relief

Are there any global hunger relief organizations that provide vegan food for the hungry?

Occasionally dilemmas arise when vegans must make a calculated choice that stretches the limits of their ethics. Fortunately, these occurrences are rare and, due to the far-reaching efforts of some highly dedicated people, hunger relief is one area where compromise is unnecessary. It's true that many charitable hunger relief organizations (such as CARE and the Food and Agricultural Organization of the United Nations) support animal husbandry projects in areas where traditional customs include this practice. However, there are two remarkable organizations that provide vegetarian and vegan hunger relief throughout the world.

VEGFAM, founded in 1963, provides short-term emergency assistance and supports finding long-term solutions to extinguishing chronic hunger, including using highly innovative and ecologically sound methods. You can write to them at The Sanctuary, near Lydford, Okehampton, Devon EX20 4AL, England, or telephone them at (011) 44-182-282-0203. The American Vegan Society (AVS) has agreed to take donations in U.S. currency and make them available to VEGFAM in British currency. Donations must be specified General or Projects Only, and checks should be made payable to American Vegan Society but noted "for VEGFAM." Write to AVS at P.O. Box 369, Malaga, NJ 08328, or call them at 856-694-2887.

The largest global plant-based food relief program is the Hare Krishna Food For Life (FFL). Their mission is to distribute vegetarian and vegan meals to the disadvantaged and victims of disaster (natural or manmade) wherever in the world there is a need. They also provide counseling, health education, and sustainable agriculture and living skills training to those in need. Food For Life established Feed the World Week (held October 15 to 21 each year), which coincides with Vegetarian Awareness Month (October) established by the North American Vegetarian Society. Feed the World Week has been observed in many countries, including Australia, Croatia, Finland, Germany, India, Taipei, the United States, and countries in South America. For more information on Food for Life or Feed the World Week, write to 10310 Oaklyn Drive, Potomac, MD 20854 or call (301) 983-6826.

My local vegetarian group is considering preparing and serving a vegan meal at a community soup kitchen. Is this a good idea?

Some activist groups volunteer a few times a year or during holidays to prepare and serve vegan meals at community kitchens and homeless shelters. Although their motives are pure, the approach is problematic. Generally no education is provided to the managers of these programs, leaving the staff completely clueless about the health and financial benefits of plant-based eating. As a result, these events do little to encourage the ongoing implementation of vegetarian meals. In addition, one-time programs place people who are desperate in the degrading position of being a captive audience. They are not making a conscious decision to be vegetarian or even to consume a vegetarian meal. It is patronizing and demeaning because they have no choice. Their needs are urgent, and their options are negligible. The activists may feel charitable about their efforts, but in the long run these experiences tend to be more self-serving than constructive.

The prevailing public attitude is that any surplus food should be suitable for the hungry and that poor people should accept what is given freely without question. Sadly, the majority of poor people are also among the least healthy and the least educated, and they have little access to information that would present an alternative perspective about animal-based foods. Unfortunately, serving vegan food a couple times a year does nothing to alter this situation.

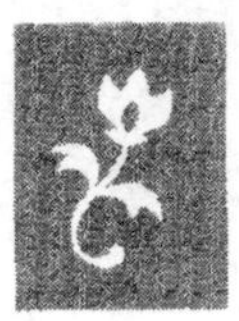

The prevailing public attitude is that any surplus food should be suitable for the hungry and that poor people should accept what is given freely without question.

A better solution would be to offer free or very inexpensive vegan cooking classes at shelters, community kitchens, or centers and churches in low-income neighborhoods. Students could join in the meal preparation, and then everyone could sit down at the table and share in the bounty of their efforts. This way people would be participating because they were genuinely interested, and they would also gain some familiarity with vegan recipes. In addition, students would leave better informed to make wiser, more healthful food choices and be empowered with valuable and practical knowledge.

Even though they do wonderful, vital work, I'm uneasy supporting local food banks, community kitchens, and shelters because they deal a lot with meat and other animal products. Any suggestions?

Most urban food banks warehouse and broker food destined for community kitchens and homeless shelters. Due to limited refrigeration and storage facilities, they tend to receive an abundance of nonperishable items including plenty of canned goods and refined carbohydrate products. This leaves food banks and kitchens clamoring for provisions that are considered more nourishing by conventional standards, such as meat and dairy products. Government-surplus foods replete with animal fat, such as butter and cheese, are highly desired and welcome. Vegan staples such as fresh vegetables and fruits, legumes (peas, beans, and lentils), and whole grains are among the most nourishing and least expensive foods available, but they are rarely on the menu at establishments that assist the hungry.

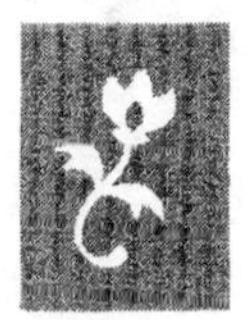

Vegan staples are among the most nourishing and least expensive foods available, but they are rarely on the menu at establishments that assist the hungry.

If you want to participate in direct action to alleviate hunger, there are many ways you can help. You can:

- purchase and donate vegan food to a food bank or give it directly to a kitchen or shelter;
- solicit vegan food donations from supermarkets, food cooperatives, and natural food stores;
- ask local farmers to plant a row of crops to donate, then arrange for pickup and delivery;
- organize volunteers to glean fields after the harvest;
- go to farm markets and ask for donations of fresh produce that isn't sold by closing;
- become involved in your local Food Not Bombs group, a grassroots network of volunteers that provides free hot vegan meals as well as social and political support to low-income people in communities throughout North America and Europe; or
- present vegetarian education programs at your local food bank.

Keep in mind that it is pointless to arrange for donations of produce or unusual foods if no one has any idea what to do with them. Also, if your donations are merely viewed as a way to stretch the animal-based items a little bit more, they will help feed people in the short run but they won't have any long-term impact.

Food has an emotional hold over all of us, including those of us who don't have much.

Grassroots education is essential if any alternative hunger relief program is going to be effective. Many people don't know much about vegetarianism and are fearful about it or simply disinterested. They may not be aware of how it might benefit them, or they may be turned off by foods that are unfamiliar or seem weird.

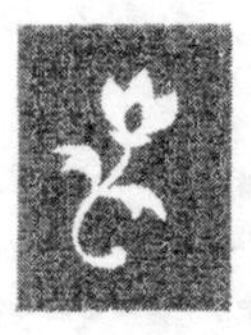

Grassroots education is essential if any alternative hunger relief program is going to be effective.

It is important to understand and respect people's cultural and ethnic differences, too, and realize that food has an emotional hold over all of us, including those of us who don't have much.

Hunger is a complex issue with manifold causes and solutions. There are a variety of avenues for vegans to help those who are less advantaged, both directly and indirectly. However you choose to contribute, your generosity and compassion will make a difference in the life of someone in need.

Veganism on Campus

I want to educate the people at my college about veganism. Do you have any ideas on how I should go about this?

It is always easier and more effective when there are a number of people behind public awareness campaigns, so organizing a group would be one of the best ways to begin. But even if you are the only vegan involved, there are still many outreach efforts you can do on your own.

Here are just a few ideas to get you started. You will probably be able to come up with many more of your own.

- Coordinate a school vegan society and recruit members by placing notices in the school paper, monthly calendars, and on bulletin boards. If there is a vegetarian society or animal rights group in your city, solicit their help.
- Prepare a library display of books and periodicals about veganism.
- Arrange a presentation by a nationally recognized speaker.
- Write an article for the school newspaper or a letter to the editor.
- Organize a vegan share-a-dish meal.
- Do an on-air interview through your school radio station.
- Distribute information on campus and outside the dining hall.
- Set up a booth at school events to hand out vegan literature.
- Host a vegan education conference.
- Coordinate a screening of vegan-related videos.
- Write and circulate a vegan newsletter.

I am a freshman in college who recently decided to go vegan "cold tofu." The dining hall is not vegan-friendly. What can I do to help turn things around?

College students are one of the fastest growing segments of the vegan population and their influence has been astounding. Due to the efforts of student groups around the country, many colleges are now offering vegan, or at least vegetarian, options at most meals.

Probably the reason these alternatives aren't being provided at your school is because the staff and administration do not see a demand for them from the student body. If you are the only person on campus who wants animal-free meals, then their rationale would appear to be justified. However, it's unlikely this is the case. Because there is strength in numbers, a group can be significantly more persuasive than a single individual. Banding together with other vegans and vegetarians on campus will give you much more leverage than you could muster alone.

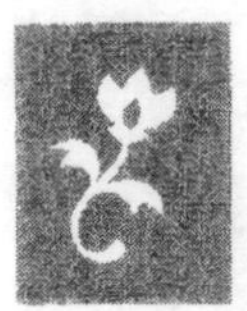

No student should be forced to sacrifice her or his ethical beliefs simply because accommodations do not exist at the present time.

Seek out other like-minded students and make the issue as public as possible to stimulate interest. Circulate a petition around campus and at the entrance to the dining hall. If you find any professors or student government members who are also interested in vegan meals, they may be able to provide additional support and lend authority and validity to your efforts.

Talk to the director of food service and express your concerns. Realize that the food service personnel probably know very little about veganism, so be patient, courteous, and understanding when you explain what vegan eating entails. Be willing to propose suggestions on how they might be able to veganize their current standards, such as using oil instead of butter, vegetable bouillon instead of meat stock, or soy protein instead of beef. Come supplied with a variety of easy vegan recipes designed for commercial kitchens (quantity recipes are available from national organizations), and volunteer to be a resource to answer questions, offer feedback, and provide fresh ideas for ongoing vegan alternatives.

Employment and Investing

I have worked at a fast-food place since I was a teenager—long before I became a vegetarian and then a vegan. My boss and the people that work there are like my extended family. The problem is that I don't feel good about working there anymore. My coworkers aren't the problem—it just feels as if I am contributing to the meat industry, and it upsets me a lot. I can't quit because my boss is the only employer who will accommodate my graduate school schedule and pay me decently. Is there anything I can do to make working there more tolerable? Everyone there knows my feelings about the food the restaurant sells, but I still feel like such a hypocrite.

The sole reason that the restaurant you work for is in business is to promote and sell animal products. There is no way around this fact. Therefore, it is not surprising that you are finding yourself more and more uncomfortable. Nevertheless, it sounds as if you have already made up your mind that staying in this job is the only practical solution for you. Depending on where you live, this may or may not be the case. Unless you take the time to seriously explore other work opportunities, you will never know if a flexible, well-paying position is available with a more vegan-compatible company.

People who choose to be vegan make a conscious decision to be aware of the suffering to which the average person is desensitized. The only way to make your present job more bearable would be for you to revert to that mind-numbing state of denial. Although veganism can be challenging and perplexing in situations like this, it is far preferable to ignoring the truth or living a lie.

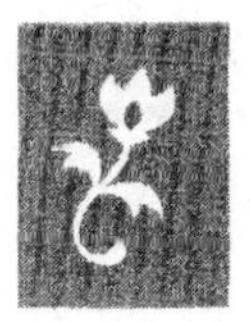

People who choose to be vegan make a conscious decision to be aware of the suffering to which the average person is desensitized.

Only you can align your life's priorities and weigh the burden this conflict bears on your conscience. Because you are so close with your coworkers and they respect you and your beliefs, they may be willing to help you network with other potential employers in your area, and your boss might be amenable to adjusting your schedule to give you time off for interviews.

If you remain in your current capacity, you will have no choice but to compromise your ethics, because there is no way to reconcile this line of work with vegan practice. If you do choose to stay because alternative opportunities are nonexistent or you determine that your need for security overshadows your convictions, you can simply remind yourself that the job is temporary. Then, as soon as you are able, look for work that harmonizes with your beliefs.

I am a vegan, but one thing that bothers me is that I work at a grocery store in a deli department. I can't afford to quit my job since I go to school, and I need money for my tuition. My salary is excellent. Is this wrong?

Vegans, like everyone else, need to earn a living. When people become vegan before entering the workforce, it is usually much easier for them to design a career path that is aligned with their convictions. However, when people embrace veganism after they have become well entrenched in a nonvegan occupation, it is much more difficult to disengage themselves and start anew.

Selling nonvegan deli items such as cold cuts, cooked meats, and cheese, and promoting or otherwise encouraging customers to purchase animal-based foods is unquestionably contrary to vegan values. Nonetheless, you are in a fortunate situation. Most grocery stores have numerous departments that would not directly conflict with your vegan ethics. Grocery stores generally sell a wide variety of vegan items, such as household supplies, fresh produce, flowers, and dry goods, so their focus is not specifically on selling meat and other animal products. It would probably be much easier to apply for a transfer to a different department than it would be to seek employment elsewhere. It is also possible that you could retain your existing salary and at the very least not have any lapse in income during the shift.

If you feel obligated to remain in your current capacity because there are no other assignments within the store and you do not want to jeopardize your finances, then you may want to temporarily stay in your present position but look for new opportunities in alternate fields during your off hours. There may even be a chance to work in a paid position related to your course of study if you take the time to explore what else is available to you.

Just because you need to work doesn't mean you must compromise your beliefs. Only you can weigh the level of discomfort you feel in this role. If it bothers you sufficiently, you will be willing to put your energies into seeking a well-paying post in a more vegan-compatible line of work.

I am trying to be responsible and educate myself about how to establish financial stability for myself and my husband. I know that the best way to put aside long-term savings for retirement is through the stock market. But none of the material I have read about investing addresses the issue I face—I want to avoid investing in companies that exploit animals. Are there any brokers or mutual funds that specialize in addressing the concerns of vegans? Do their funds do reasonably well, or are my husband and I better off just stashing our money in the mattress?

How and where we invest our money can have a significant impact on social change in addition to affecting our personal finances. Socially responsible investing (SRI) is the catch-all phrase for integrating one's values and societal concerns with investment decisions. The notion of SRI grew out of the interests of religious institutions that wanted to screen out investments in alcohol and tobacco. The concept evolved in the 1960s and '70s when issues about war, nuclear weapons, nuclear power, civil rights, and women's rights raised awareness among investors. Objections to apartheid in South Africa in the 1980s further solidified support among institutional and private investors. In the 1990s, environmental considerations attracted attention, stimulating investments in "green" companies. Today's top concerns are the environment, social justice, fair and nondiscriminatory labor practices, health, and animal welfare.

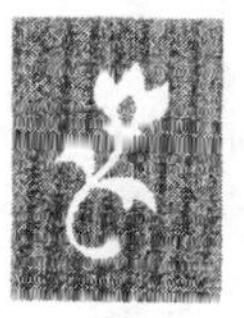

Humane investment strategies encourage companies to take account of the social and environmental costs of doing business.

Financial advisors who specialize in socially responsible investing are scattered throughout the United States. They are well versed about this ever-changing field and are best equipped to help you determine the wisest options for your particular needs. As with any financial decision, it is invariably prudent to discuss your needs with an experienced and knowledgeable professional you can trust.

In the past twenty years, socially responsible mutual funds have expanded tenfold. Many of these types of investments do quite well but, as with any financial venture, there is always an element of risk. You and your husband will need to ask for and study the prospectus of each company, fund, or product to determine its suitability in light of your values. You will also want to discuss its history, stability, and potential return on your investment with your financial advisor.

Before seeking socially responsible investment practitioners, products, or services from organizations primarily devoted to SRI, be sure to ask about the ownership and commitment of the parent company or affiliated organization. In some cases, they may not have socially responsible investing as a priority. Also, some SRI products may not be vegan-friendly, even though they may be advancing positive change in other ways.

The influence of responsible investing is evident locally and globally, directly and indirectly. Your humane investment strategies will help encourage companies to take account of the social and environmental costs of doing business and foster an economy that works for the planet and all its inhabitants.

Animal Concerns and Activism

I have been learning more and more about the endless atrocities done to animals, and I am so anxious to help! I want to bring awareness to people and help understanding spread throughout the world. What can I do to get involved?

The atrocities perpetrated by humans against animals exceed all horrors that humans commit against themselves, both in kind and quantity. Animals have no recourse against us, no means of escape, and no way to fight back. They are vulnerable and completely at the mercy of our species. For many vegans, this defenselessness makes the plight of animals a priority over all other forms of suffering. This doesn't imply that vegans cannot and do not work to alleviate human travails concurrently; they often do. Rather, it means that vegans tend to reach out first to those individuals with the greatest need and the least resources.

The animal activist population is small, but the number of animals in distress is incalculable. It is for this very reason that you must carefully assess your ability to commit to the long haul before taking action. So often eagerness turns to apathy when activists discover that progress and personal reward are disproportionate to the efforts expended. Burnout and depression can easily set in, especially when we realize that the abominations so evident to vegans are virtually invisible to the public at large.

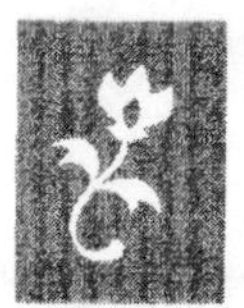

The atrocities perpetrated by humans against animals exceed all horrors that humans commit against themselves, both in kind and quantity.

Be selective and pace yourself. Choose only one group or project to work for initially and plan to devote a predetermined amount of time to it each week. There are countless animal issues to pick from, so try to get involved with one that sparks your passion. You can function independently, start up or join a local group, or work for a national organization. There are advantages and disadvantages to each, so it really comes down to a matter of personal style. Grassroots efforts can be very powerful and offer the benefit of knowing the area and audience you are trying to reach. In addition, working locally allows you to directly survey the impact of your actions. Determining what to do will depend on your interests, time, and talents.

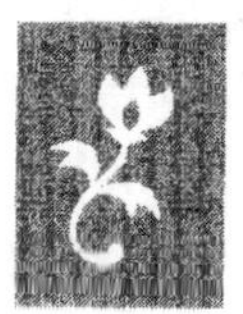

Animals have no recourse against us.
They are completely at the mercy of our species.

Because vegans are so keenly attuned to the suffering in the world, it is tempting to try to do everything all at once to stop it. Unfortunately, this is not only ineffective, it can be enervating. It is disheartening to be aware of flagrant atrocities while simultaneously acknowledging our limited ability to relieve them. Nevertheless, this is necessary to maintain sanity in the face of such depravity. It is also essential to preserve balance by nourishing your spirit in positive, joyful ways. Exposing oneself constantly to misery can be stifling, so occasionally take a breather away from it to refresh your perspective, clear your mind, and simply have fun.

The animals need you. Give what you can, as much as you can, as often as you can. But don't forget to enjoy your own life while you are working to save the lives of others. Whenever your arms reach out to embrace the animals, make sure you wrap them around yourself now and then, too.

I'd like to educate others about the exploitation of horses. Please advise.

Horses are used by people for a variety of purposes: entertainment (such as circuses, parades, and rodeos), monetary gain (such as race-track gambling), labor (such as farming, ranching, packing loads, pulling weights, and transportation), display (such as competitions and shows), and personal pleasure (such as riding and camping). For each of these circumstances, the appropriate stock is essential. Therefore, superior breeding is a top consideration and stud services are highly profitable enterprises.

The majority of horses that do not exhibit the desired characteristics, become ill or injured, or are past their prime are killed. It is just too costly to maintain an unproductive animal, so, for a horse, being put out to pasture typically means a grueling trip to the slaughterhouse.

The horse trade is a covert and intricate business network that is often brutal but extremely lucrative. Concerned vegans can work in a variety of ways to help alleviate the suffering and needless death of horses. Here are a few ideas:

- public education through presentations, leafleting, and letters to the editor
- boycotting and leafleting at local racetracks
- protesting circuses, rodeos, and other entertainment venues that use horses
- writing articles for newspapers, magazines, or other publications
- working to enforce legislation that bans or regulates racetracks
- adopting retired racers, work horses, or other breeds, if the appropriate space and facilities are available

I raise and ride horses. Is this considered nonvegan? I can understand why bull riding and activities of that nature are wrong, but I don't know about this one.

Much of the natural landscape that was once home to many wild animals, including horses, no longer exists. It has been demolished for the sake of our ever-burgeoning human population and to appease our seemingly endless desire to turn the beautiful earth into a concrete jungle. Many of the once-free animals that were forced into human servitude have no habitat to which they could return even if they were released. In addition, after centuries of domestication, these animals have become virtually dependent on humans for their survival.

Most people whose lives include animals are enriched and rewarded beyond measure. This is because domestic animals, in general, accept and love humans unconditionally. Despite our differences, we are able to develop amazing relationships that transcend the confines of our distinctions.

It is hard to imagine that such seemingly respectful and reciprocal alliances could in any way be harmful or exploitative. Yet when animals are bred, raised, and sold to be used for racing, work, entertainment, or human pleasure, the innocence of the relationship is sullied.

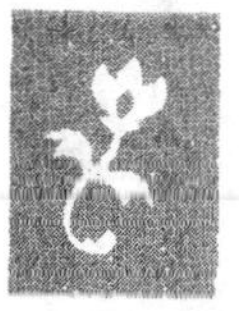

Veganism does not view any living being as a commodity.

Rescuing and nurturing abused horses is a noble activity. However, breeding horses for sale, regardless of how kind and loving their care may be, is not considered a vegan occupation. This is because philosophic veganism does not view horses—or any living being—as a commodity. Regarding a life as "stock" or "merchandise" reduces it to the status of possession, justifying manipulation and misuse for profitability.

Certainly, domestic horses need to be exercised, but if they are used for human indulgences, it only reinforces the misperception that animals exist to serve people. This belief, known as *speciesism,* is comparable to both racism (i.e., black people exist to serve white people) and sexism (i.e., women exist to serve men). From the wholly compassionate perspective of veganism, none of these views is acceptable.

Vegans who adopt a horse (regardless of whether or not money is exchanged) have in essence made an ethical promise to attend to that animal's health and well-being for the remainder of her or his natural life. Tame horses that are unable to run free need exercise, and extending loving care obligates you to provide that exercise, which typically involves riding. Adopting a horse in need is not the same as breeding or acquiring horses for status, financial gain, or work. Nevertheless, riding, grooming, and caring for horses can be personally gratifying and fosters mutual joy and friendship that transcends the barrier between species.

My beloved dog died a few weeks after I became vegan, and my family wants to get another dog. We used to put our dog in a cage occasionally when we left the house for several hours so that she would not urinate in the rest of the house. I don't want to do this anymore, but my mom says that dogs don't mind these cages. I can't see how caging an animal we love and leaving him for hours at a time isn't cruel, even if the dog just spends the time sleeping. Can caging companion animals be considered ethical if there is evidence that it is not unpleasant for the dog? What can I say to my mother to convince her not to do this?

You have my deepest condolence for the recent loss of your dear companion. In an ideal world, no animals would be kept at all by people, let alone indoors or in cages. Sadly, our present world is far from ideal, and often concessions are necessary to achieve a higher objective.

Because we are concerned about and accountable for the health and safety of our companion animals, human guardians are obligated to take certain precautionary measures. This includes obtaining licenses and tags for dogs and attaching them to a collar around each dog's neck. To comply with ordinances and to prevent accidents from occurring, human caregivers fasten leashes to these collars or to harnesses when dogs are outdoors. Dogs are bathed and groomed, given vaccinations and other inoculations, dipped in flea deterrents, housebroken, have their nails trimmed, and are trained to respond on command. Most of the deeds done to dogs are not only in the dog's best interest, they are in the human's best interest as well, if not more so. In many instances, these acts are essential for the humans and canines to peaceably co-exist.

Some people would simply refuse to adopt a dog if they thought the animal would damage their home or belongings. Although most people who take in dogs are genuinely committed to and love their animal companions, their feelings are usually contingent on whether the dog complies with their standard of acceptable behavior. A dog who urinates in the house after puppyhood is rarely tolerated.

Most dogs endure being caged, after a period of adjustment. As long as it is only for short intervals, there is access to food and water, the enclosure is large enough for the dog to move about, stand up, and turn around, and it is in a secure, shaded location, caging should not do the dog harm. Of course, it would be best if human companions could stay with their dogs throughout the day and night, but most people work or leave their home now and then, so for the vast majority of folks this is not feasible. Sometimes it comes down to the choice of adopting a dog and caging her at times or not adopting at all. In the face of this very real scenario, many more dogs would remain homeless or be euthanized, a far worse prospect than temporarily being caged.

It may be difficult to accept your mother's point of view, but until you have your own living space, you–and any dogs you adopt–must observe her stipulation. Brief caging is not in and of itself injurious. By protecting the house and safeguarding the dog in this way, you will be helping to save a life that might otherwise be forsaken.

Uninvited Intruders

Is there a vegan way to control ants? We usually get infested every summer.

Sugar ants, commonly called the derogatory name "piss ants," are difficult to control. What they lack in size they more than make up for in population and persistence. In turn, it requires tenacity and patience to banish them from your home.

Keep your house immaculately clean. Pay particular attention to the kitchen and dining areas. Empty garbage daily and store it in tightly sealed trash cans away from the house. Do not leave food of any kind open or out, including items destined for the compost heap. Store sugar and other sweeteners in sealed, airtight containers, and store liquid sweeteners in the refrigerator. Wipe the outside of jars and keep them clean and dry. Thoroughly rinse out bottles and cans before recycling them. Scrub countertops frequently, taking care to clean under (not just around) small appliances. Do not let crumbs accumulate on the countertop, floor, or in or on furniture. Sweep regularly and often. Remember, a particle of food is a feast for an ant; a small amount more can sustain a colony for many days or even weeks.

Keep your kitchen and bathroom dry. Wipe out the sink, tub, and shower after each use. In many cases, ants are in need of water as much as food.

If you have companion animals, place their food in a moat. Take a bowl slightly larger than their normal dish and fill it with water. Then place the food dish in the water-filled one. Although ants need water to live, they don't like to swim.

Seal up all observable cracks and potential points of entry around the infested area. Use a caulking gun designed for indoor purposes. This is not only helpful in controlling ants, it will help to keep out other unwanted insects as well. In addition, sprinkle paprika, cayenne, peppermint, or talcum powder where the ants enter your home and, in the garden, scatter powdered charcoal around your plants. This will deter the ants without harming them.

Bees have built a nest in the wall of my house. What can I do?

Before deciding on a solution, it is helpful to positively identify the specific type of insect you have: yellow jackets, wasps, hornets, bees, or mud daubers. Not all stinging insects are aggressive or necessarily dangerous, unless you or someone in your family is allergic to their bite or sting.

It is hazardous to remove occupied nests unless you fully understand the nature of the inhabitants and what needs to be done to avoid serious harm. If the insects pose a direct threat, it may be necessary to call in a professional. In some areas there are professionals who specialize in the nonchemical removal of nests of certain types of stinging insects such as yellow jackets. The collected nests are then sold to pharmaceutical companies that make antivenom from the dead insects. As an alternative, you can request that they relocate the nest to a wooded area or field. Of course, if you find a professional willing to provide this service, there would most likely be an additional charge.

Stinging insects have a short life cycle, and cold weather generally kills off the colony. If the nest does not present a clear danger, you may want to leave it alone and simply let nature run its course.

We just returned from some traveling and discovered that our house had a lot of activity in it while we were gone. There were mouse droppings all over our kitchen counter! Yuck! What should we do?

Chances are that you have more than one mouse. Set several humane, box-type, releasable traps (available at most hardware stores, humane organizations, and through specialized mail-order catalogs) and check them frequently. Peanut butter is a popular lure, but a piece of dry breakfast cereal is less messy and just as effective. Once caught, mice become very frightened and, because of their high metabolism, they can get hungry and thirsty very quickly. When you find one in the trap, release her or him at least 50 to 100 yards from your home, or further. You can always take the captured mice in the car with you and release them a mile or so away. If you release them too close to your home, they will undoubtedly find their way back.

Mice need food, water, and shelter, and evidently they found them at your home. Here are some important tips to keep in mind to discourage a future invasion:

- Make sure all water faucets are turned off and none are dripping. Wipe off the area around sinks and countertops and check to make certain they are dry.
- Make sure all potential entry holes are plugged or sealed. Most mice that get into homes are very tiny and can fit through astonishingly small openings.

- Make sure that absolutely *no food* is accessible to them. In other words, put *all* your flours, grains, cereals, crackers, cookies, bread, pasta, sugar, and so on in airtight containers, canisters, or jars. Mice can smell quite keenly and have surprisingly sharp teeth.

If your home is free of easy-to-get food and water and the entry holes are closed, the mice won't return. Well, they may come back once or twice (if they can get in), just to check and see how good a job you've done trying to keep them out. If you've done your homework, they'll move on.

Clothing, Shoes, and Outerwear

Are there other materials and fabrics besides leather and wool that aren't vegan? How can I determine what to avoid?

The skin, fleece, feathers, shells, hair, or body parts of any animal, bird, fish, or insect are not vegan. This includes fur, down, silk, camel's hair, mohair, angora, tortoiseshell, fish scales, snakeskin, ivory, bone, pearls, and so forth. The list of animals and their body parts used for human garments and accessories is extensive. When shopping, just use your common sense and don't purchase something if you don't know its origin. There are many vegan alternatives for practically all these animal-based commodities; for example, faux pearls, rayon or tencel instead of silk, synthetic fiberfill instead of down, polar fleece instead of wool, and taugua nut instead of ivory.

Now that I've become vegan, what should I do about the nonvegan clothing I already own? I'm not too keen now on wearing it. I'd have to wonder what kind of message I would be sending as a self-proclaimed vegan in wool, silk, or leather shoes. Hypocritical at best, I fear.

Virtually every new vegan encounters the dilemma you are presently facing. Often it is not easy to part with nonvegan items for a variety of reasons. Finances are a critical consideration, because even though the heart may be willing, if the wallet is empty new purchases will be forestalled by necessity. It is important to weigh the odds: What is your comfort level wearing nonvegan items now that you have made an ethical commitment to veganism? How long will it take for you to save enough money to replace essentials, such as shoes, that are nonvegan? Do you already own vegan alternatives that you could use in the meantime, even if they aren't ideal?

You are correct in thinking that wearing animal products would appear disingenuous and could easily send a distorted message about veganism to others. To avoid wastefulness, some vegans wear their old nonvegan items only in the seclusion of their own home and put on their "veganwear" when they are out in public. This addresses the issue of frugality on two levels: utilizing what is already owned and extending the life of one's vegan products through prudent use. However, many vegans find wearing animal-based commodities to be ethically and emotionally excruciating, and they cannot bear to don them even in private. Consequently, each vegan must determine her or his own threshold of tolerance and make choices based on individual need and economic circumstance.

There are many creative and practical ways to dispose of animal-based commodities such as yard sales, consignment shops, thrift stores, shelters, or gifts to nonvegan friends or relatives. Some vegans donate the proceeds from the sale of their nonvegan items to animal rights organizations; others use the profits to purchase vegan replacements.

If you feel you cannot part with your prevegan commodities right now, then hold onto them until you are prepared to let them go. When you are ready, you will be able to devise imaginative and serviceable ways to discard them. Releasing these final remnants can be an incredibly liberating experience, filled with the satisfaction of no longer needing to justify apparent conflicts of conscience.

I know that one reason cited for people not wanting to wear or use leather items they acquired before becoming vegan is that it sends the wrong message to others. But what about fake leather clothing or shoes that look like leather? Should vegans actively try to avoid the appearance of nonvegan products?

Some vegans do not want their clothing, shoes, outerwear, or accessories to be mistaken for their animal-based counterparts and therefore prefer apparel that is not leatherlike in appearance. Others feel that because synthetic look-alikes are harm-free, there is nothing problematic with wearing them. Vegans occupy all strata of our society, and those who function in mainstream positions often prefer to blend in and not draw attention to themselves or their personal philosophies. Synthetic leathers can help them do just that.

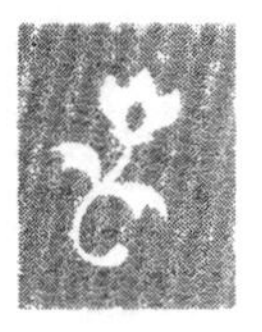

Vegans do not have to sacrifice fashion or function to enjoy conventional attire.

Another benefit of wearing imitation leather is that when nonvegans inquire about a vegan's shoes, belt, jacket, wallet, briefcase, gloves, and other articles of clothing with regard to one's ethical consistency, it can be very enlightening to point out that these items are indeed synthetic. Most nonvegans are unaware that today's mock leather is comfortable, breathable, flexible, and durable. They frequently are surprised to discover that vegans do not have to sacrifice fashion or function to enjoy conventional attire.

I was shocked to hear about the way wool is obtained, and I would like to know of some cruelty-free fabrics that will keep me warm instead.

Polar fleece is a terrific alternative to wool. It is lightweight, not bulky, quick drying, hypoallergenic, breathable, long-lasting, and cruelty-free. In addition, a number of manufacturers use recycled materials in their polar fleece, making it an excellent green product. To obtain maximum warmth, polar fleece should be layered with other articles of clothing. A way to thwart the wind is to wear a nylon shell over polar fleece. The shell adds no weight and serves double duty as a light outergarment in milder weather. There is even specially made windblock fleece material that prevents cold air from penetrating the fabric. Outerwear made from this material is extremely versatile and can be worn as a single layer.

Jackets and coats stuffed with synthetic down or fiberfill provide excellent warmth without bulk or added weight. Some are available with a specially treated shell that makes them both windproof and waterproof. Polar fleece hats and scarves abound and are very cozy. You can also find accessories made from woven acrylic or cotton, although they do not provide as much insulation as polar fleece. Woven cotton sweaters come in a wide variety of colors and weights and, when layered with a shirt or turtleneck top, they can keep a person mighty toasty. Finely woven microfiber, microsuede cotton, and corduroy slacks, blazers, and sport jackets are available in a range of weights and wale sizes. Once again, layering will help to further block out the cold and wrap you in warmth.

I'm shopping for cotton pants and finding virtually everything is now "prewashed for softness." I'm aware that most commercial fabric softeners are animal based, made from tallow. Is there a way to buy all-cotton clothing that hasn't had an animal bath? Or is this one of those unavoidable vegan compromise situations?

If we thoroughly dissect the cotton clothing industry, we will discover many important factors that could be of concern to vegans. For instance, cotton is typically grown in fields saturated with chemicals and pesticides, creating hazardous run-off, dangerous working conditions, and damage to the earth. Picking and collecting cotton inadvertently injures or kills small animals and insects. If cotton is bleached, the process adds carcinogenic dioxins to our land and water supplies. Hauling cotton requires transporting it in trucks that pollute our air and contribute to global warming. The tires of trucks contain animal byproducts and the roads they use caused destruction of habitat and native plant species and displaced wildlife when they were built. The majority of employees at the plants where cotton is spun and woven into fiber eat meat and wear leather shoes. The factories where the clothing is sewn utilize equipment that, at the very least, requires animal-based lubricants. In addition, many articles of clothing are made in sweatshops in other countries where the labor force, which often includes children and minors, works painfully long hours in filthy conditions for dastardly owners who pay a pittance for wages. Finished items must be transported to various stores and warehouses or are promoted in catalogs that don't used recycled paper and that contain images that were photographed on gelatin-based film.

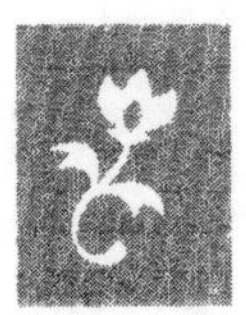

The key to vegan sanity is to refrain from microanalyzing and to realize that aiming for perfection is counterproductive.

So, is cotton vegan? Yes, as much as anything can be vegan in our modern world. This is not necessarily a compromise. It is a matter of being realistic in light of the resources available to us. It is easy to get mired in the technicalities of vegan living. But, if we scrutinize the components of practically any commodity, we will undoubtedly discover something in its development or processing that is animal-based or otherwise nonvegan.

The key to vegan sanity is to refrain from microanalyzing, accept that vegan purity is unattainable, and realize that aiming for perfection is counterproductive. This does not imply that we toss in the towel and give up. It merely means that we must realign our priorities and focus on the bigger picture if veganism is to have any meaningful and lasting effect.

The alternatives for wool and leather all seem to be made from petroleum products like synthetic fleece and plastics, often made by large chemical companies with questionable ethics. The petroleum and chemical industries are responsible for much suffering, environmental destruction, and poor use of resources as well. Is there a clear ethical choice?

Animals do not have a closetful of clothing; what nature provides is all they possess. For humans to expropriate an animal's skin, fur, fleece, or feathers, they must deny its basic needs and ultimately take its life. Every piece of animal-derived apparel represents a minimum of one and often multiple lives that have been needlessly sacrificed for human indulgence.

Every day, more and more vegan alternatives become available because there is a growing demand for them. While the situation is not yet ideal, reasonable replacements for leather and wool do exist. Synthetic leathers are flexible, sturdy, breathe, and preserve all the functional qualities of animal hides without the carnage. Although a few large corporations produce a preponderance of these products, several small start-up companies make fantastic vegan "leather" shoes and jackets, and some manufacture their goods from vegan recyclables, making them more environmentally sound as well as practical. The same is true for polar fleece articles, which can be spun from recycled plastics and other reusable items. In addition, these products are durable, so they seldom need to be replaced.

Layered cotton and corduroy and synthetic fleece-filled outwear lend weightless warmth. Nylon, vinyl, rubberized cotton, and other treated fabrics guard against the elements without forfeiting ethics. It is true that petroleum-based products are not exemplary, but they are not the only option in many situations. When they are, the key is to buy infrequently and make the items currently owned last as long as possible.

Leather and wool are the direct result of willful, premeditated slaughter. Harm caused to animals by petroleum-based goods is ancillary because it is not the primary motivation of the industries that produce them. The distinction is intention as well as repercussion. Both the leather and plastics industries wreak environmental havoc, but only one aims its artillery at an individual's head.

I've heard that silk screens are used to print T-shirts. Wouldn't this make the T-shirts nonvegan?

Silk screening is a printmaking technique in which color is forced through the pores of transparent mesh cloth that is stretched over a heavy wooden frame. Traditionally, silk or fine organdy muslin was used. Today silk is very costly and with a variety of less expensive, high-quality substitutes readily available, few artists, if any, use it. Polyester is currently the most popular fabric used for silk screening because it is both durable and affordable. Silk-screened T-shirts are vegan.

Personal Care and Health-Related Products

When a product is tested on animals, what exactly does that connote? Does it mean the product was tested when it was first made but not any longer? Do companies test products periodically or only when they change a formula?

When companies test personal care and cosmetic products on animals, they may test one, several, or all the ingredients. In addition, they may test the combined group of ingredients that comprises the final product. Once a product has been tested there is no need to test it again unless the formulation has been changed. Because manufacturers regularly develop "new and improved" products, those who conduct animal tests have a never-ending rationale to continue to do so.

Some manufacturers will state that they do not test their products on animals and, technically, this may be true. However, they may contract out to other companies to do their testing for them, or they may use ingredients that have only recently become available and have undergone testing elsewhere. Other companies may have tested their products on animals at one time but have discontinued the practice because they have not introduced any new products or formulations.

There is no government mandate requiring personal care and cosmetic products to be tested on animals. Companies that have never performed animal tests–on their premises or contracted out–usually use ingredients that were tested on animals many years ago or those that are generally regarded as safe.

I am looking for cosmetics and personal care products that are vegan. Some companies tout the fact that they don't do any animal testing, but then they still put animal-based ingredients in their products. How can I tell if something is "clean"?

Because there is no legal definition for the term cruelty-free, manufacturers are able to take liberties with its interpretation and use. Shortly after the expression was popularized in the United States, it became clear that listing cruelty-free on a product label was an effective selling tool and an excellent way to garner consumer confidence and loyalty.

Unfortunately for shoppers, companies that narrowly construe the phrase to mean simply that a product has not been tested on animals—with no regard to whether or not the product contains animal-based ingredients—cloud the issue. Of course, this makes finding truly cruelty-free products more difficult.

Adding to the confusion, several well-meaning organizations have created cruelty-free logos for companies to incorporate into their packaging. The problem with this approach is that the determination of the ethics of a company, product, or product line is based solely on the manufacturer's word, and not on any third-party investigation or outside confirmation. This is not because these organizations feel this is an unimportant task. However, they are generally tightly budgeted groups that lack the time, money, and staff necessary to perform independent certification services.

A number of products found in natural food stores are labeled "no animal testing and no animal products (or by-products)." Often these are good choices, but it is still wise to read the ingredient list or call the manufacturer's customer service department to inquire about any questionable items and explore the source of ambiguous ingredients.

Are there alternatives for vitamins in vegan casings? Several of my current ones are in gelatin capsules.

Gelatin capsules are almost always made from animal gelatin, the protein extracted from the tissue of steers, calves, or pigs. Vegetable-based gelatin capsules are becoming more popular, not only to meet the demands of vegans and vegetarians but also to satisfy the requirements of certain religious groups. The capsules, which are free of all animal by-products and preservatives, are derived from chemically inert vegetable cellulose. Most manufacturers that use a vegetable gel cap feature this information prominently on their product labels because it is a valuable sales tool.

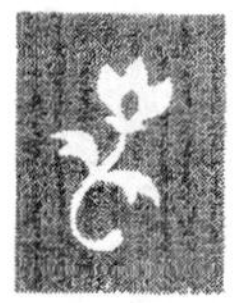

The purchase of gelatin products directly contributes to the support of the animal by-products industry.

A small number of specific supplements are currently available only in animal-based gelatin capsules. If you have no alternative but to use a supplement with this type of delivery system, you can separate the capsule and mix the contents with a food or beverage, or, in the case of an oil, you can squeeze the contents out of the capsule and onto a spoon. Do this for each capsule just before using.

Even if vegans do not ingest a gelatin capsule directly, the purchase of gelatin products still contributes to the support of the animal by-products industry. If you have no other options at this time, and doing without the supplement would cause you suffering or harm, then by all means take it. The vegan ethic invokes you not to put your health in jeopardy. Encourage manufacturers to switch to vegetable-based gelatin capsules, and support those that already do. But in the meantime, do what is necessary to maintain your health while striving to eliminate the broader aspects of suffering for both humans and other animals.

I was wondering if there is a safe, effective method of birth control that is not tested on animals. I have eliminated all animal products from my diet, purchase only cruelty-free products, and am opposed to vivisection, yet I feel like a hypocrite because I continue to take birth control pills. Are there any birth control methods that are cruelty-free?

Practically all pharmaceutical products have been tested on animals, are derived from animals, or contain animal by-products. This includes most birth control drugs and devices. For instance, lactose (milk sugar) is a standard excipient (an inert substance that forms a vehicle for a drug). It is used in most pharmaceutical tablets, including birth control pills. In addition, pharmaceutical companies routinely conduct research on live animals for new or altered drugs. Consequently, all birth control drugs are the result of studies that included animal subjects and are produced by companies that are involved with vivisection. Although a few brands of condoms are vegan, most condom manufacturers test product coatings on animals and the spermicides and lubricants may contain animal products.

Surgical sterilization (for you or your partner) is another option. However, it is critical to be absolutely certain prior to undergoing sterilization that you do not want to have children, because it is a permanent choice. Although these surgeries can sometimes be reversed, such procedures can be painful, difficult, and costly, and are not always feasible.

Natural birth control is an excellent, drug-free method, but it requires a significant commitment from both parties. For natural birth control to be effective, a woman must be able and willing to take and record her basal body temperature at the same time every morning; inspect, interpret, and record the characteristics of her vaginal secretions; and chart the course of her ovulation and menstrual cycles to determine fertile and infertile intervals. The male partner must be willing to abstain from sex during the woman's fertile times throughout the month. Both must accept that sexual relations may be less than spontaneous. It is also very helpful if the woman has a regular menstrual cycle and is in a stable relationship, and both parties have a strong desire to avoid pregnancy.

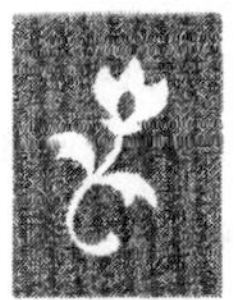

We need to make the best choices we can based on the world we have inherited, not the society we envision and are trying to create.

Unfortunately, there are no birth control methods available at this time that are suitable for all people and are safe, effective, hassle-free, and vegan. You must weigh the alternatives against the consequences of having an unwanted child and determine the method that you and your partner are most comfortable using. If the decision comes down to a less-than-perfect birth control method versus an unwelcome pregnancy, the compassionate option is to avoid the potentially disastrous situation by employing prevention.

We need to make the best choices we can based on the world we have inherited, not the society we envision and are trying to create. Making concessions for birth control is not indicative of hypocrisy. It simply means that you are being realistic, practical, and responsible.

Everyday Commodities

I recently read a meat industry piece that claimed that plastics are produced in part from animal by-products. If this is true, it leaves me wondering about polyester, vinyl, and other animal fabric substitutes. Could you shed some light on this?

Plastics refer to any group of synthetic or natural organic materials that can be molded, cast, extruded, drawn, or laminated into films, filaments, or objects. The production of various plastics entails a complex chemical process that typically includes petroleum along with many types of resins, resinoids, polymers, cellulose derivatives, proteins, and casein materials. Casein, a regenerated protein derived from cow's milk, may be combined with formaldehyde to form casein-formaldehyde. It may also be combined with rennin, an enzyme obtained from the stomach lining of animals, to create rennet-casein.

These animal by-products are not used in the manufacture of all plastics and, when viewed as a percentage of the whole, they comprise an infinitesimal part of the constituents used in the overall production of plastics. Thus, the financial bearing these by-products have on the animal slaughter industries is negligible and essentially inconsequential. Because there are no perfect alternatives for every animal-based item, vegans must choose to tread as lightly as possible by selecting the most compassionate choices available. The amount of animal ingredients used in some plastics is trifling when compared with true animal commodities, such as leather, wool, or down, which directly fuel the continual slaughter of animals.

As vegans, we must confront the fact that our world, our options, and even our own actions are fallible.

As much as we may want to be fastidious in our elimination of animal-based commodities, there are realistic considerations that make this impractical. From the perspective of compassion, economic impact, and the ability to inspire change and create a demand for genuinely humane products, our present-day substitutes, despite their drawbacks, are far superior to commodities that represent obvious suffering and death.

What should vegans do about candles? Beeswax ones are not vegan, but I have health and environmental concerns about using paraffin. Are there any alternatives?

Nearly all candles on the market are made from paraffin wax and animal fats, except for a small number that are made from beeswax. Nevertheless, even beeswax candles are often a blend of beeswax and paraffin because beeswax is several times more costly. Paraffin candle wax is made from the residue collected from gasoline refining. It was developed more than 150 years ago when the petroleum distillation industry was launched and needed a way to dispose of excess sludge. When paraffin candles are burned, they release black petroleum carbon soot deposits. These are carcinogens known as *petro-soot,* and they are considered as harmful as secondhand tobacco smoke. This is problematic from both a health and an environmental standpoint.

Fortunately, candles made from pure plant waxes are becoming more readily available. You can generally find them in natural food stores, specialty gift shops, or through mail-order suppliers. These all-vegetable candles come in a variety of elegant colors and styles, including tapers. Some are even designed for use with aromatherapy and are scented with vegan essential oils.

Is ink that is used in pens, markers, books, and other printed matter vegan? If not, what's a vegan to do about such ultra essential things?

Ink is generally made from complex synthetic dyes, resins, solvents, and, more recently, soybean oil. Any animal derived products used in inks would be infinitesimal and essentially inconsequential to vegan practice.

It is fruitless to stew about microscopic quantities of nonvegan materials that may or may not be in our everyday essentials because, if you look hard enough, chances are you will find them in practically everything. Brooding about incidental ingredients that require a doctorate in chemistry to comprehend detracts from the essence of compassionate living and turns it into an obsession that has little to do with vegan philosophy or reverence for life.

When the source of by-products is eradicated (i.e., meat, eggs, and dairy), the by-product industry will cease to exist. In the meantime, focus on avoiding obvious animal-derived ingredients and, in addition, accentuate personal acts of kindness, generosity, and gratitude that will more readily inspire and hasten the caring world vegans envision.

Chapter 4

Vegan Practice and Food

Feeding the Heart

A pervasive myth that has persisted for years is that vegetarians are intrinsically more kindhearted than their meat-eating counterparts. This is founded on two basic misconceptions: (1) Gentle people are intuitively attracted to a meatless diet, and (2) a meatless diet naturally makes aggressive people more gentle. The underlying assumption is that food has a strong influence on personality or that personality dictates tastes. Neither is accurate. Although certain foods (such as sugary sweets, refined carbohydrates, chocolate, and caffeinated beverages) and those to which we are allergic or sensitive can affect *mood* and *demeanor*, our basic *character* is not molded by the foods we eat. Dietary patterns and food preferences are influenced primarily by culture, ethnicity, availability, familiarity, custom, convenience, taste, mood, and economics. Food, in and of itself, doesn't change our values or the core of our basic nature.

There is no evidence that vegetarians are more sensitive or magnanimous than anyone else. History is scarred by the acts of monstrous vegetarians as much as it is filled with the contributions of selfless others. To assume that diet alone could shape one's character is to ignore a wealth of psychological and sociological factors that have a much tighter grip on our principles, personality, and palate.

People are drawn to vegetarianism for a multitude of reasons. Although some people have referred to vegetarianism as a social movement, it is absurd to think that a cultural revolution could be fashioned by a group whose eating habits have elements in common but whose ideologies are incongruous. Veganism, on the other hand, encompasses significantly more than what one eats or doesn't eat. It includes a "reverence for life" philosophy exhibited through tangible endeavors in all areas of daily living, making it a far more tenable route to effect social change.

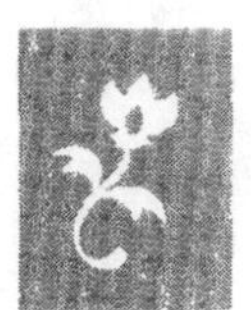

Compassion is an affair of the heart and spirit; it has little to do with the head and even less to do with the stomach and mouth.

Social reformation instigated by compassionate individuals is essential for producing a compassionate culture, not to mention a compassionate world. Food choices alone won't do it. Transformation requires a fundamental shift in priorities, and veganism can provide not only the rationale but the tools. However, is becoming vegan sufficient to induce compassion?

There are three principal reasons why people adopt a vegan lifestyle: (1) to do as much as possible to eradicate suffering in the world, (2) to generate inner peace by eliminating conflicts of conscience, or (3) to expunge karma by observing religious proscriptions. (Karma is a doctrine espoused by a number of Eastern religions, including Buddhism, Jainism, and Hinduism. It teaches that every thought and deed creates its own effects, which must be endured or enjoyed by the individual concerned. Karma also relates to reincarnation and one's ability to ascend to enlightenment. Negative karma will impede such advancement. However, negative karma can be counterbalanced or overcome by engaging in acts of kindness and compassion.)

The desire to end suffering in the world may be based on intellectual realizations and not necessarily on altruistic empathy. Also, if individuals are motivated toward veganism solely for reasons of personal gain, such as inner peace or karmic relief, it would not be accurate to say they are driven by compassion. Nevertheless, it is true that when people strive for peace, whether it is internal, external, or spiritual, they are less likely to engage in actions that would inflict suffering on others, even though their justification might be that doing so would in turn impose suffering on themselves.

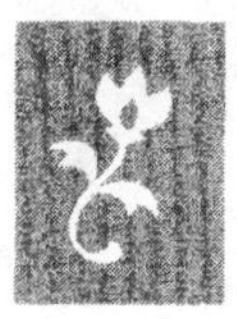

To become wholly compassionate we must force ourselves to look directly into the face of suffering. Only then will we see our reflection and know that the hurt of others is equal to our own.

A compassionate disposition is cultivated. It is not the osmotic result of what one eats or even what one does. It is the consequence of a conscious and concerted commitment to awaken to the suffering around us, and then caring enough to do whatever is necessary to end it. This awareness begins with a longing to see the truth. It is not rooted in erudite theories or abstract concepts. It is not a question of whether a cat or a dog or a fish or a cow or a pig or a person feels pain and suffers, and certainly not a matter of degree or impressive statistics. All we need to do is open our eyes, our ears, and our hearts, and the truth will flood our being with compassion.

Even once we perceive the anguish of others, it is tempting to turn away. Empathic people have tender spots that can be frightening and overwhelming to acknowledge. But to become wholly compassionate we must force ourselves to look directly into the face of suffering. Only then will we see our reflection and know that the hurt of others is equal to our own.

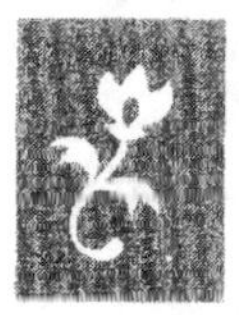

A compassionate disposition is not the osmotic result of what one eats or even what one does. It is the consequence of a conscious commitment to awaken to the suffering around us.

Compassion is based on faith, not fact–faith that others feel and suffer as we do. This point was unequivocally confirmed and powerfully driven home by the severely mentally challenged populations I worked with for many years. Although they did not have a deep capacity for intellectual analysis, they were among the most loving, caring, sensitive, and genuinely empathic individuals I have ever known.

Compassion is an affair of the heart and spirit; it has little to do with the head and even less to do with the stomach and mouth. Neither food nor rhetoric entertain compassion. Fostering compassion merely necessitates paying attention, noticing every moment of our lives, every thought and every deed, and doing the most in each moment to alleviate suffering and promote harmony, justice, and peace.

Vegans are not inherently more loving, generous, kind, or thoughtful than nonvegans. However, vegan precepts do present a pragmatic structure for nourishing and guiding our compassionate nature, independent of whether veganism or compassion comes first.

Even though vegan practice deals with much more than what one eats, diet seems to be its primary distinguishing feature. This is where the majority of people begin their journey to veganism, and for many it is the most exciting aspect of vegan living. Because eating is typically something we do three times a day or more, and it is an activity that gives us great pleasure, food holds an important place in our psyche and our hearts. When shifting to veganism, people usually place their initial focus squarely on their diet. Regardless of culture, ethnicity, or country of origin, new vegans are always interested in and fascinated about vegan cuisine. Learning what is and isn't vegan, figuring out how to plan meals, exploring unusual foods, and discovering new ways of cooking and eating are all part of the adventure.

Clarifying and Transitioning

What does a vegetarian eat that a vegan does not? Are vegetarianism and veganism very similar except that vegans do not eat dairy products?

There are a number of distinctions between veganism and vegetarianism, but the primary difference is the totality involved in vegan practice, which includes much more than diet alone. This makes it difficult to compartmentalize individual components of a vegan lifestyle, because veganism considers all aspects of behavior as interrelated.

Among the many ways that vegans manifest their reverence for all life is by choosing foods that are exclusively plant-based. Both vegans and vegetarians eschew the obvious products of death in their diet—meat (of any color), fowl, and fish. However, vegans and total vegetarians (people who abstain from animal products in diet only) go several steps further by avoiding all other foods of animal origin, such as eggs and animal milk products, which are less conspicuously brutal but in reality are equally as gruesome as meat. Vegans also do not consume honey or foods that were processed with or contain animal by-products.

Among the many ways that vegans manifest their reverence for all life is by choosing foods that are exclusively plant-based.

Except for these additional parameters, the foods that vegans and vegetarians can choose from are the same. Some people approach plant-based eating from a health perspective and therefore elect to follow a dietary plan expressly designed to improve their physical well-being. As a result, some vegans may observe a fish-free macrobiotic diet, a natural hygiene system, a raw foods program, or take some other tack that has nothing to do specifically with being vegan. These diets are merely individual approaches to what some people consider to be healthier ways of eating. They do not reflect any general guideline to which vegans as a group are obliged to comply.

Because veganism's underlying impetus is one of compassion, not health, it is certainly possible to find vegans who do not eat an overly well-balanced or wholesome diet. Others, of course, may be particularly concerned about eating healthfully. Like all groups of people, vegans have different tastes, quirks, habits, and interests. Their food choices, although always plant-based, reflect their diversity.

At the present time I am an ovolacto vegetarian, but I am interested in becoming vegan. Do you have any suggestions on how to make the switch?

Many vegans start out as vegetarians, and this is a great way to transition to a totally plant-based diet and lifestyle. Begin by taking an inventory of the animal-based products that remain in your life. Then decide whether you want to first revise your diet, focus on other aspects of vegan living, or do both simultaneously. To change your diet, determine which animal-based foods you most rely on, and investigate the vegan alternatives that are available.

It is not hard to find appropriate foods to eat if you know what you should be looking for. Every mainstream supermarket stocks hundreds of items that are vegan, even though they may not be labeled specifically as such. Vegetables, fruits, juice, beans, rice, bulgur, cornmeal, flour, pasta, tomato sauce, tomato paste, salsa, bean dip, nuts, seeds, hot and cold cereal, bread, jams, jellies, peanut butter, applesauce, soups, pretzels, bagels, tortillas, popping corn, pickles, relishes, and many canned and frozen items are vegan. From these foods alone you could devise an amazing variety of meals and snacks. In addition, you may also find specialty products such as tofu, nondairy milk, meat analogs, and vegan frozen desserts–all this without taking a step inside a natural food store! But, if you do go to a natural food store, you'll find an extraordinary selection of even more vegan choices.

From a dietary perspective, the only difference between vegans and vegetarians is that vegetarians may use dairy products, eggs, and honey, and vegans don't. Your choice as you become vegan is to simply eliminate these foods or find suitable options. The stronger your commitment is to making the change, the easier and more enjoyable you'll find the passage.

I'm currently trying to figure out the difference between vegan and macrobiotics. They seem very similar. Why would one choose a vegan lifestyle as opposed to macrobiotics?

Macrobiotics is an Asian dietary system based on the ancient Chinese philosophy of yin and yang. It is designed to promote good health, vitality, and longevity through a diet largely based on whole grains and a lifestyle that fosters healthful practices. Macrobiotics does not include animal foods except for fish and fish products, which are optional.

Macro means *big,* and *bios* means *life.* Hence, macrobiotics is the pursuit of a "big life," in quantity as well as quality. Most people who practice macrobiotics are not vegan, even if they forego fish. This is because macrobiotics is a predominately health-based system, so there is no incentive for practitioners to eschew animal products in clothing or other commodities. Veganism, on the other hand, is a lifestyle based on the ethic of compassion. This principle infuses all aspects of a vegan's life; diet is merely one element of how the vegan tenet is expressed.

Some vegans choose to follow a fish-free macrobiotic diet because they believe it is health-supporting and personally beneficial. Nevertheless, there is no direct connection between macrobiotics and veganism. Vegans as a group practice a wide variety of eating styles and many alternate among an assortment of approaches.

What would a typical vegan meal be?

There is so much diversity that there really is no typical vegan meal. Often new vegans just replace their old animal-based foods with cruelty-free versions and analogs. Others explore the vast range of vegan ethnic cuisines and incorporate a variety of foods from different lands and cultures. Some vegans eat quite simply, centering meals around whole grains, beans, and vegetables; others are attracted to gourmet dishes and exotic specialty foods. There are clusters of vegans who practice a fish-free macrobiotic diet, or a "living foods" (mostly raw) diet, or a fruitarian diet. And, of course, there are those who fluctuate among all these approaches and maintain continual variety.

The beauty of vegan eating is that there are no rules and no need to follow the antiquated pattern of meat, potato, and vegetable. Hence, being vegan can open the door to a world of unlimited culinary possibilities.

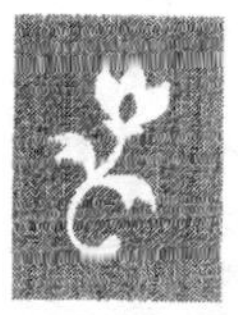

Vegans practice a wide variety of eating styles and many alternate among an assortment of approaches.

Many vegans claim they never ate so well or with so much pleasure before becoming vegan. With certain foods off limits, vegans tend to become more open and creative with their meal planning and more willing to try new foods. In essence, each meal becomes an adventure, an opportunity to experiment with unusual ingredients and seasonings and a chance to test innovative ideas. A vegan meal can be as plebeian as a hearty soup with crusty rolls or as sophisticated as delicate pastries stuffed with imported mushrooms and savory smoked tofu.

All vegans have a different tale to tell about their favorite styles of eating, and the potential combinations are endless as well as exciting. The typical vegan meal begins and blossoms in each cook's imagination.

I am a nineteen-year-old female who wants to become vegan. What are some basic foods I should stick with until I get the hang of it and stop needing meat?

Everyone approaches veganism in different ways. Some people dive right in and make the transformation overnight; others need a little more time to test the waters. If you are highly motivated, you can get the hang of it just by looking through the endless recipes in the many vegan cookbooks available and perusing the wide variety of fresh, packaged, and frozen foods at your natural food store.

There is no physiological requirement for meat, so your need for it is purely psychological. Fortunately, there are innumerable products available today that help make the shift from omnivore to herbivore pain-free and delicious. They also take the brainwork out of meal planning, especially for those who are used to placing meat at the center of their plate. Meat analogs have proliferated, including plant-based products that simulate ground beef, turkey, chicken, ham, bacon, sausage, pepperoni, burgers, nuggets, hot dogs, cold cuts, and more. In fact, for most people on the road to veganism, giving up meat is perhaps the easiest change to make for a number of reasons: (1) It is a healthful switch; (2) meats can only be disguised so much; it's generally fairly obvious that meat is the flesh of a cadaver and that "juice" is a pseudonym for blood and body fluids; and (3) chewy, flavorful, cruelty-free alternatives abound.

Most supermarkets carry an array of meat analogs that appeal to those who want to thwart heart disease as much as those who don't want to eat body parts. One of the most beautiful aspects about these foods is that budding vegans who have an emotional attachment to familiar styles of eating can now have their "meat" and stomach it, too.

Fiction, Fact, and the Unexpected

I am trying to lose weight. I have been vegan for three months and have lost just a few pounds since then. I'm discouraged but not giving up. Any pointers?

A vegan diet is just one part of a vegan lifestyle and was not designed to be a weight-loss program. Although, on the average, vegans and vegetarians tend to be a bit slimmer than omnivores, and many find it easier to maintain their ideal weight, there is no magic tool for knocking off the pounds. It is a myth (albeit a hard one to eradicate) that all vegans and vegetarians are lean. Poor lifestyle and dietary habits can proliferate among vegans and vegetarians as readily as they do among meat-eaters. You can still be a vegan on a diet of greasy potato chips, peanuts, and nondairy ice cream!

Research continually points to a low-fat, well-balanced diet that includes plenty of fresh fruits, vegetables, and whole unrefined grains, combined with regular daily exercise, as the best route for achieving and maintaining one's ideal weight. A good diet and exercise plan work in synergy and do not provide the same health-supporting benefits independent of each other. Moreover, diet alone is frequently insufficient for achieving long-term weight loss. Therefore, in addition to evaluating what you are *eating*, take a look at what you are—or are not—*doing*.

Some physicians who promote a whole foods, plant-based diet do not feel that the quantity of food is the primary issue in weight loss, but rather the kind of food that one consumes. For the vast majority of people, there is no need to put any limit on fruit and vegetable intake. In fact, most health care practitioners and dieticians encourage eating significantly more of these foods than the general public currently consumes. Whole unprocessed grains and beans can also be eaten with little restriction by most people. These unrefined, natural whole foods are packed with flavor and nutrition while containing virtually no fat and few calories.

Where problems start occurring is when processed and refined foods are introduced into the diet. These foods tend to contain high amounts of fat, including harmful trans-fats; large amounts of sodium, which is not only unhealthful but causes water retention and bloating; and little to no fiber, which adds bulk that fills us up, not out.

Often, people eat unconsciously. In other words, they eat while doing other things–such as watching television, driving, sitting at the computer–and are unaware of how much food they are putting in their mouths. Typically, they are munching on processed snack foods, chips, cakes, cookies, soda pop, or candy. Analyze your eating and snacking habits to see where you might be adding unnecessary fat and calories to your diet and displacing more wholesome foods. You may be very surprised to discover what foods your diet is centered around and what other foods you've consumed very little of. This will help guide you to the foods that need to be increased in your diet and those that should be drastically reduced or omitted.

If you have other weight-related concerns or health problems, be sure to consult your physician or health care practitioner before starting a rigorous change in diet and exercise. If you need more in-depth information relating to your individual nutritional requirements, contact a nutritionist or dietician who is familiar with vegan diets. This way she or he can tailor your diet and meal plans to meet your special needs.

Why do vegans eschew animal products but use plant-based foods that epitomize animal products, such as fake cheese, veggie burgers, veggie sausages, and so forth? Even though they are not actually animal products, I refuse to use them because of what they represent.

Most people aren't raised as vegans (at least not yet, at any rate), so adopting a totally plant-based diet can pose some very real challenges. The standard American diet is centered around animal products, and it is hard for some people who want to practice a compassionate lifestyle to reorient their thinking about this. Few new vegans are well acquainted with alternative foods and different styles of eating, so vegan cheeses, veggie burgers, and meat analogs can serve a valuable purpose by filling the void on our plates. Consequently, they can make transitioning to an animal-free diet simple and painless.

In addition to easing the task of meal planning, these foods appease our emotional and psychological attachment to particular flavors and textures. Even though analogs are not the real thing, they are similar enough to provide a sense of familiarity. They assuage cravings for commonplace comfort foods and old standbys that are truly products of cruelty and death. When vegans eat these foods, they know that they are made from plant sources, not animal parts, so there is no deception involved. At the same time, these foods satisfy tastes that many of us are accustomed to and were raised to enjoy. They also allow vegans to partake of corresponding American favorites that nonvegans consume—burgers, hot dogs, ice cream, and more—without sacrificing their values or harming others. Furthermore, analogs are generally quick, easy, and fun to prepare.

Most vegans do not view fake meat, cheese, and dairy products as explicit replacements for their animal-based counterparts but as delicious foods in their own right. After all, most meats are pretty bland without adding seasonings and condiments. Vegan alternatives simply incorporate some of the herbs and spices that are used to flavor prepared meats, since this is what vegans miss most—the flavors, not the meat itself.

There is nothing harmful or embarrassing about indulging in vegan alternatives, and it is inaccurate to think that vegans who eat analogs are suppressing a longing for animal-based foods. Analogs may resemble meat, eggs, or dairy products in many ways, but they have one significant difference—they are animal-free.

I've heard that yellow food dyes come from pigs and that common red food colorings contain beef blood. Is this true?

According to the U.S. Food and Drug Administration, the organization that approves and regulates food, drugs, cosmetics, and their additives in the United States, all food colorants are derived from plant, mineral, or synthetic-organic compounds and are not obtained from animal sources. The only exception is the red dye cochineal, also known as carmine, which is derived from the dried and ground bodies of the female cochineal insect. Most food products that contain cochineal or carmine should have them listed as such (not as a numbered dye) on the ingredients label. Although the rumor persists that other food dyes are animal-derived, they are, in fact, vegan.

I heard that animal products are used in the manufacture of alcoholic beverages. Is there any truth to this rumor? If so, how can I be sure that my beverage is safe?

Certain alcoholic beverages, such as wine and beer, typically go through a clarifying or fining process to remove impurities and improve their cosmetic appearance by making them clear. Although earth-based agents, such as bentonite clay or activated carbon, may be used, particularly with less expensive brands, animal-derived agents are commonly employed, especially with more costly European wines. These include egg whites, whole milk, casein, gelatin, or isinglass (made from the bladder of sturgeon fish). Isinglass is used predominately by German wineries, although other European and a few American wineries also use this substance. Wines from some Mediterranean countries may be clarified with the blood of large mammals; however, this process is prohibited for use with wines produced in the United States and has been banned by the European Union since the 1997 mad-cow disease scare.

Kosher wines produced in the United States are less likely to have been clarified with animal-based agents, but there is no general rule. Each certifying agency may use different criteria for what is permissible, so a kosher symbol is no guarantee that a particular wine is vegan.

You can contact individual manufacturers directly to investigate. However, many companies use processes that they consider to be proprietary, or they may alternate among agents depending on market prices. Consequently, companies may be reluctant to attest that any particular product or procedure is vegan.

The clarifying and fining agents used in the filtration of wine and beer are relatively minute (for instance, two to three egg whites can clarify approximately 55 gallons of wine; 1 ounce of gelatin can clarify 1,000 gallons of wine), and they are not part of the finished product. So can alcoholic beverages that have been clarified with animal-based agents be considered vegan? This is a controversial issue, similar to the concern about bone char filtration that is sometimes used in the production of cane sugar.

When viewing wine and beer (and, indeed, *all* our foods and beverages) from a compassionate perspective, there are several additional issues to be weighed. Foremost is consideration of the laborers who gather the grapes and other key ingredients. Are they treated well, fairly compensated, and protected from exposure to pesticides and other toxins? Are the beverages organically produced, using sustainable, nonpolluting methods? Do you consider these beverages essential to your health and well-being? Are substitutes for these products available to you?

Some vegans avoid alcoholic beverages entirely, believing that they are addictive, cloud the mind, dull the senses, numb the heart, and impede our ability to make wise and compassionate choices. Others eschew alcohol because of religious proscriptions or personal health concerns, or to avoid excess caloric intake. On the other hand, some vegans find the effects of alcoholic beverages to be pleasurable, believe that in limited quantities they can be health-supporting, and appreciate the flavors they impart in cooking.

The decision to use or not use alcoholic beverages is a personal one. Nevertheless, there are many options available to vegans who want to avoid them, such as dealcoholized wine and champagne and nonalcoholic beer in a variety of brews. And, of course, there are always fruit juices, fruit juice blends, sparkling water and cider, and chilled herbal teas.

I have been a vegetarian for over a year now and am beginning to pursue my beliefs a step further into veganism. The only obstacle I am finding is that many of the ingredients in foods are animal products or by-products in disguise. Can you provide a list to help me identify the most common animal products used that I wouldn't otherwise recognize?

A number of ingredients often found in commercially produced food products are typically animal based and easily identifiable. A few of the most common are albumin, calcium caseinate, calcium stearate, carmine, casein, cochineal, gelatin, honey, isinglass, lactase, lactose, lard, myristic acid (tetradecanoic acid), oleic acid (*cis*-9-octadecenoic acid), palmitic acid (hexadecanoic acid), pancreatin, pepsin, propolis, royal jelly, sodium caseinate, suet, tallow, and whey.

What complicates matters is that many ingredients that appear to be animal derived could have been made from plant sources or produced synthetically. Some of these are adipic acid (hexanedioic acid), capric acid (decanoic acid), clarifying agents, disodium inosinate, diglyceride, emulsifier, fatty acid, glyceride, glycerol, lactic acid, magnesium stearate, monoglyceride, natural flavoring, polysorbate, sodium stearoyl lactylate, and stearic acid. Often manufacturers don't know if their ingredients are from animal or nonanimal sources, because buyers frequently alternate among suppliers, depending on who has the lowest market price. In other words, there may be no definitive way for you to determine the origin of certain ingredients.

Many people who are new to veganism get caught up in an endless and frustrating search for hidden animal ingredients. Some vegans become consumed to the brink of obsession with unearthing the tiniest trace of animal derivatives. Sadly, this misses an integral point of being vegan, which is to reduce suffering. Instead, these vegans end up chasing rainbows and ultimately heap anguish upon themselves and those around them.

Abstain from buying, using, or supporting any commodities, ingredients, or enterprises that are obviously and incontrovertibly nonvegan. However, avoid striving for personal perfection at the cost of realistic and achievable goals. By accentuating the attainable, you will release yourself from needless anxiety and will help make compassionate living more appealing and practical to nonvegans, thus advancing the vegan cause.

Reading Labels

Exactly what are those "natural" and "artificial" flavors that are added to processed foods?

"Natural" and "artificial" flavors often are not explained on package labels because many companies consider certain product information to be proprietary. These additives may be derived from plant, animal, or synthetic sources. To verify the origin of flavorings in specific products you will need to contact the company directly. Many manufacturers have toll-free numbers direct to their customer service departments, and most will be pleased to provide this information.

The only way to know with certainty what is in our food is to buy items that are as close to nature as possible. Unfortunately, when we purchase foods that have been processed and refined, we are at the mercy of the manufacturer.

What do the kosher symbols on the front of food products stand for, and which ones mean that the product is vegan?

The "U" or "K" symbol on a product means that it is certified kosher. Kosher means that the item was prepared in accordance with *kashrut* (Jewish dietary laws), under the supervision and approval of a certifying organization and rabbi. It does not indicate that the food is vegan, as animal products may also be labeled as kosher.

"Kosher parve" denotes that the food is deemed *neutral,* which means that it does not contain meat or dairy products. Nevertheless, *kashrut* does not interpret *meat* in the same way that vegans do. For instance, fish and eggs are considered parve, so prepared foods marked as "kosher parve" may contain either or both of these as ingredients.

A "D" means that the food is designated "kosher dairy." That is, it is certified kosher but it contains dairy products or derivatives and, in accordance with *kashrut,* must not be eaten with meat. "DE" signifies that the food does not contain dairy products directly but was prepared on equipment that also is used to make foods containing dairy. In terms of *kashrut,* these foods are considered kosher dairy, even though the equipment is thoroughly cleaned before each run and the product itself is dairy free.

A kosher symbol on food does not imply that it is vegan. Kosher certification merely ensures compliance with ritual animal slaughter and certifies that meat and dairy products have not intermingled during processing. There is no direct correlation between kosher foods and veganism.

Are there any commercially produced whole-grain breads that are vegan?

Vegan breads abound in all varieties, from Italian rolls to Essene bread to whole-grain buns to bagels, pita, chapatis, tortillas, lavosh, and more. Small bakeries often have a few vegan items among their options, as do many well-stocked supermarkets. The most wholesome and widest array of vegan breads, however, can be found in natural food stores. The commercially produced breads that most supermarkets carry frequently contain dough conditioners, colorants, chemicals, or preservatives. Although many of these ingredients may be vegan, they are unnecessary additives that health-conscious consumers generally avoid.

Wherever you purchase your bread, be sure to read the ingredient label carefully. Frequently used nonvegan ingredients include, among others, eggs, milk, milk powder, whey, butter, and honey. The easiest way to determine with certainty that a bread is vegan is to look for simple ingredients that are easily recognizable and clearly understood. Avoid buying breads with ingredients that are confusing or do not sound like real foods.

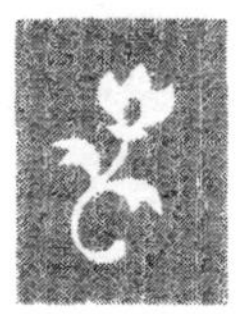

To determine with certainty that a bread is vegan, look for simple ingredients that are easily recognizable and clearly understood.

Basic yeasted bread requires just a few ordinary ingredients: flour, water, and yeast. Nevertheless, it is common to find a few other items added to vegan breads, such as sweeteners, salt, herbs, or vegetable oil. They add flavor, impart richness, create a finer crumb, improve texture, or promote a higher rise.

Most pita breads, plain bagels, chapatis, corn tortillas, and lavosh are vegan, but always check the ingredients to be sure. Flour tortillas are often vegan, but some brands contain lard, which is an animal fat. Some brands of crackers may also contain lard, butter, milk derivatives, or cheese. Many commercially produced baked goods, including breads and crackers, contain cottonseed oil or hydrogenated fats, which are vegan but not very healthful.

Finding vegan bread is not difficult. In fact, bread in all its forms is one of the more readily available vegan foods. The secret is to look closely at ingredient labels, ask questions, and seek out the highest quality product made with comprehensible ingredients.

Could you please tell me about casein? I am trying to be dairy-free, but when I purchase rice or soy cheese, casein is listed on the ingredient label. I was told it is dairy. Is it?

Yes, casein is a dairy derivative. It is a protein found in animal milk that is added to a number of commercial cheese substitutes to improve their texture and help them melt better. Although some brands do not contain casein, it is wise to read product labels carefully since manufacturers sometimes change their recipe formulations or switch ingredients without notifying consumers. Also, when you go out to eat, be sure to ask about any soy cheese products before placing your order. Many restaurants that offer vegan options unwittingly replace dairy cheese with soy cheese that contains casein. Most servers and even chefs do not know that casein is derived from cow's milk, so it would be a great opportunity to check out the product label and enlighten the restaurant personnel.

Puzzling Foods

What is yeast, and is it vegan?

Yeasts are single-celled microscopic organisms which, as they grow, convert their food into alcohol and carbon dioxide through a process known as fermentation. Yeast is used by winemakers, brewmasters, and bakers in the making of wine, beer, and bread. The carbon dioxide from yeast is what makes beer frothy and champagne bubbly and causes yeasted bread dough to rise. Pure yeast, regardless of the strain, is vegan.

To multiply and grow, yeast needs moisture, food (in the form of sugar or starch), and a warm, nurturing environment. Wild yeast spores are constantly floating in the air and landing on uncovered foods and liquids. They are used to promote the natural fermentation of certain foods such as sauerkraut and pickles and provide the leavening for breads that traditionally do not contain added yeast, such as sourdough bread.

The Egyptians used yeast as a leavening agent more than 5,000 years ago, and fermented beverages, including wine, were made for thousands of years before that. Scientists have been able to identify and isolate specific yeasts that are best suited for various purposes. The principal yeasts used today are baker's yeast, brewer's yeast, and nutritional yeast.

There are a number of different types of baker's yeasts, but all are considered alive, that is, active and capable of leavening bread. Brewer's yeasts are special nonleavening yeasts used in the manufacture of beer. Brewer's yeast that is sold in natural food stores is a by-product of the brewing industry. Because it is a rich source of B vitamins, it is often promoted as a health food, but brewer's yeast can have a very bitter taste and is not recommended for use in cooking. Another product commonly found in natural food stores is torula yeast, which is a nonleavening yeastlike organism that is grown on waste products from the wood pulp industry.

Brewer's yeast and torula yeast are frequently confused with nutritional yeast. Nutritional yeast is a primary grown food crop, which means it is cultivated specifically for use as a nutritional supplement. This yeast is dried at higher temperatures than baking yeast, rendering it inactive. Unlike the live yeasts used in breadmaking and brewing, nutritional yeast has no fermenting or leavening power.

The brands of nutritional yeast I recommend are Red Star Vegetarian Support Formula, found in the bulk food section of natural food stores, or KAL nutritional yeast (which is repackaged Vegetarian Support Formula), available in canisters. These are currently the only nutritional yeast products with a consistent nutritional profile that is rich in the B-complex vitamins riboflavin, niacin, thiamin, and biotin, and includes a reliable source of vitamin B_{12} (cobalamin), an important nutrient often lacking in vegan diets. The B_{12} used in these products is derived from natural bacterial fermentation, not animal products, and their careful growing process ensures a high-quality source of protein with essential and nonessential amino acids. These nutritional yeasts also contain folic acid, which is important for the formation, growth, and reproduction of red blood cells, and provide several minerals including selenium, chromium, zinc, phosphorus, and magnesium.

In addition to its use as a supplement, nutritional yeast adds a delicious nutty flavor to many foods. Its chameleonlike qualities make it highly adaptable, and it is prized by vegans for its uncanny ability to add poultry-, egg-, and cheeselike undertones to vegan dishes.

Some individuals who have difficulty digesting yeasted or fermented foods often find they have no problem tolerating nutritional yeast. Nevertheless, people who are allergic to yeast should avoid all the various types of yeasts and abstain from products that contain them or that have been fermented.

How is vinegar made, and is it vegan?

The word *vinegar* originated from the French *vin aigre,* which means "sour wine." Vinegar starts with a fermented liquid such as wine, beer, or cider, to which special bacterial strains are introduced. Bacterial activity then converts the liquid into a weak solution of acetic acid, which we know as vinegar.

There are many different varieties of vinegar that are popular today. All are considered vegan.

- *Apple cider vinegar:* A fruity vinegar made from fermented apple cider
- *Balsamic vinegar:.* A sweet vinegar made from white Trebbiano grape juice, aged for many years in wooden barrels
- *Brown rice vinegar:* A mild, mellow vinegar made from fermented brown rice
- *Distilled white vinegar:* A harsh tasting vinegar made from grain alcohol
- *Fruit vinegar:* Made by blending soft fruits such as peaches, blueberries, or raspberries with a mild vinegar; sometimes sugar or fruit liqueurs are added to enhance flavor and offset acidity
- *Herb vinegar:* Made by soaking one or several different kinds of herbs, such as tarragon or dill, in white or red wine vinegar or apple cider vinegar
- *Malt vinegar:.* A mild vinegar made from malted barley
- *Umeboshi plum vinegar:* A bright, tart, salty vinegar made from the liquid used to pickle umeboshi plums, a Japanese condiment

- *Wine vinegar*:. Made from red or white wine; the flavor ranges from sweet to pungent

Are the bacterial cultures found in food vegan? What are they, and what purpose do they serve?

Bacteria are all around us–in the air, in our water, and on our food. We generally think of bacteria as pathogenic, but some bacteria, called "friendly bacteria," are considered beneficial. Certain bacterial strains are even prized and cultivated for specific medicinal and culinary purposes. For instance, some bacteria are used to produce cobalamin (vitamin B_{12}). Others are used to ferment particular foods such as yogurt, tempeh, and vinegar. It is believed that the chemical change caused by the enzymes produced by these bacteria can make foods more digestible as well as more flavorful.

Bacterial cultures are widely used throughout the food production industry. Although nonvegan foods may contain bacterial cultures, the cultures themselves are considered vegan.

What is *rhizopus* culture?

Rhizopus (also known as *Rhizopus oligoporus*) is a type of fermenting culture used to make *tempeh* (pronounced TEM-pay). Tempeh is a vegan food made from split and hulled cooked soybeans and grains that are combined with the *rhizopus* culture and incubated. The result is a firm soybean cake that is covered with an edible white mold.

Tempeh has a distinctive taste, somewhat similar to mushrooms. It is excellent steamed, baked, or pan-fried. Tempeh's succulent, chewy texture makes it an ideal substitute for meat in dishes like tacos and stew, and, when it is grated, tempeh can easily replace ground meat in traditional recipes like chili. Tempeh can also be marinated and then grilled like a burger.

Rhizopus is similar to the type of friendly bacteria used to make yogurt. However, unlike acidophilus and other cultures used to make yogurt, tempeh products should not be consumed raw. They must be fully cooked before eating to avoid stomach upset. This is because the *rhizopus* culture grows very quickly in a warm environment and, unless thoroughly cooked at a high temperature, it will continue to grow after consumption.

Some tempeh products are fully cooked and ready to use, and the directions listed on the package should contain information to this effect. Tempeh that is not precooked should be exposed to high heat for at least 20 minutes before eating.

I can't figure out whether dark chocolate or semisweet chocolate are vegan. Do manufacturers add milk?

Unadulterated chocolate is marketed as "unsweetened chocolate," "baking chocolate," or "bitter chocolate." Standards in the United States require that unsweetened chocolate contain 50 to 58 percent cocoa butter, which is vegan. When sugar, vanilla, and lecithin are added to unsweetened chocolate, the result is either bittersweet (also called dark), semisweet, or sweet chocolate, depending on the quantity of sugar used. Bittersweet chocolate must contain at least 35 percent chocolate liquor; semisweet and sweet chocolate contain between 15 to 35 percent. Adding dry milk to sweetened chocolate creates milk chocolate.

There is nothing that restricts manufacturers from adding small amounts of dry milk, whey, or other dairy products to bittersweet, semisweet, or sweet chocolate. Some chocolate makers add these ingredients to create a creamier texture and mouth-feel. Because there is no regulation regarding the addition of these ingredients, some brands of dark chocolate may contain dairy products, even though most do not. The only way to be certain is to read the package label, or you can contact the manufacturer directly if you have specific questions.

I have a Jewish friend who insists that kosher gelatin contains no animal products because it is kosher parve. Is this true?

Gelatin is the collagenous protein derived from the bones, cartilage, tendons, sinews, lips, feet, head, skin, and other connective tissue of steers, calves, or pigs. It is found in many commonplace products such as marshmallows, commercial baked goods, puddings, jelled desserts, confections, juices, roasted peanuts, sauces and salad dressings, pharmaceutical capsules, photographic film, and many hair and nail products. About half the gelatin produced in the United States comes from slaughtered veal calves.

Kosher and kosher parve are not synonymous with vegan. Kosher implies strict adherence to *kashrut*, Jewish dietary laws that forbid the intermingling of meat and dairy products. It also refers to the ritual slaughter of sanctioned animals in accordance with these laws. *Kashrut* is an ancient religious practice and is not based on the healthfulness, ethicalness, or purity of food. It deals solely with what Jewish law contends is animal, dairy, or neutral; permissible foods and their combinations; ritual slaughtering methods; and the preparation and serving of food. Thus some foods, such as certain gelatin products, may be considered parve but not vegan because, according to the laws of *kashrut*, the product has been so adulterated that it no longer constitutes meat.

As a rule, if an ingredient is listed as gelatin, it has come from an animal source. Most kosher jelled dessert mixes are made from a sea vegetable called carrageen (also known as Irish moss) or from locust bean gum (from the carob tree). Nevertheless, the only way to be certain a kosher jelled dessert is made with a vegan jelling agent is to read the ingredients list on the package.

Going Shopping

I grew up with very poor eating habits, but now as a new vegan I want to take action to replace my bad habits with more healthful ones. The problem is, when I go to the natural food store to shop, I end up completely overwhelmed. How do I work toward a balanced way of eating when all of this is so new to me and I'm not used to including many vegetables in my daily diet?

When you go to the natural food store, focus on finding the least processed organic foods and try to ignore the convenience items. Start with the organic fruit and vegetable aisles and fill up your cart with familiar produce that you know you will like. If you aren't sure which foods are the most nutritious, just use your eyes to guide you by looking for densely colored fruits and vegetables and selecting those that are in season. Try to include at least one new vegetable and one raw (uncooked) fruit or vegetable in your menu every day. This way, by the end of a week you'll have sampled seven new vegetables and they will no longer seem unusual. If one new item a day is too hard for you, try one or two new ones every week or so.

Next, go to the grain section and choose a few whole grains. When you get home, transfer them to jars with tight-fitting lids so they will be protected from moisture but you can still see them. Rice is an excellent and filling staple. You can pick from brown, basmati, wild, or a combination. Other grains you could try are millet, barley, bulgur, spelt, kamut, and quinoa.

Center your meals around a starch such as potato, sweet potato, or pasta, or a whole grain. For example, for breakfast you could have hot oatmeal or another porridge, or whole-grain cold cereal with fresh or dried fruit and enriched nondairy milk, or a whole-wheat bagel or whole-grain toast with fruit-sweetened jam and fresh fruit. Dinner could be a baked potato, steamed broccoli, and a salad. Or rice and sautéed vegetables. Or soup, salad, and whole-grain bread. Or pasta with tomato sauce and steamed greens. These are not unusual foods, but they are certainly vegan. The idea is to liberate yourself from thinking that a meal has to revolve around the meat and instead think about creative ways to include the most satisfying and healthful plant foods.

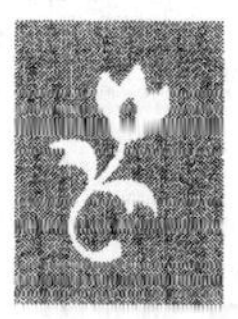

A large percentage of the convenience items found in natural food stores are no more health-supporting than the refined products available in mainstream supermarkets.

And don't forget about beans—there are so many to choose from. You can cook them up yourself (for the greatest variety), or you can purchase canned beans. It's a good idea to keep several cans of beans on hand at home so they're ready to heat and eat, add to soups or salads, or blend into dips or spreads in case you're not up to doing much cooking.

If you want to buy a few packaged items, look for those with the fewest and most understandable ingredients. Try to stay clear of anything fried or overly processed, including chips, crackers, cookies, cakes, other baked goods, and snack foods. A large percentage of the convenience items found in natural food stores are no more health-supporting than the refined products available in mainstream supermarkets. The main difference is that they cost a whole lot more. Stick with the most wholesome, unadulterated, organic foodstuffs you can find, and you won't have to worry about compromising your ethics or your health.

Are organically grown fruits and vegetables better than conventionally grown produce?

Organic fruit and vegetable farms help to maintain agricultural integrity by eliminating chemical-dependent farming practices that deplete the soil, quell biological diversity, foul waterways, decimate wildlife, harm workers, and poison the food supply. This is because organic foods are produced without the use of synthetic pesticides, herbicides, or fertilizers. Instead, organic farmers foster the earth's vitality through soil conservation and renewal, crop rotation, and the use of natural fertilizers and pest control methods. The result is cleaner, untainted produce; uncontaminated soil, air, and water supplies; and a safer environment for workers.

From a vegan perspective, however, organic farming is not perfect. Organic farms typically use a variety of by-products from the animal slaughter industries including dried blood, bone meal, manure, and other animal-derived soil enhancers and enrichments. A method of organic farming that does not employ animal-based commodities is called *veganics,* a term coined by English author Geoffrey L. Rudd in the 1940s. Veganics utilizes a variety of well-proven, widely accepted, non-animal-based organic farming techniques, such as composting with pure vegetable matter and natural pest control through complementary planting. Veganics is safe, sound, and prudent and can be implemented in small-scale home gardens as well as large commercial farms.

There is some debate over whether or not organically grown fruits and vegetables are more nutritious. Some reports state that organic produce is more nutrient-dense, but others debunk this notion. It is reasonable to assume that organic seeds cultivated in rich, vigorous soil would develop into the most health-supporting vegetation. But even if the nutritional analyses were parallel, organic (or preferably veganic) produce is more health-supporting for the earth and its nonhuman inhabitants, which is reason enough to favor it.

Is coffee vegan?

Technically speaking, all coffee is vegan. It is blended and ground from the roasted unripened fruit of a small tree known as the coffee plant.

Coffee is vital to the economies of more than fifty tropical countries. The two largest producers of coffee today are Brazil and Colombia. Coffee plantations also abound in other South and Central American countries, Cuba, Hawaii, Indonesia, Jamaica, and several African nations. Growing and tending coffee plants involves handpicking the fruit; discarding the thin, parchmentlike covering; and cleaning, drying, grading, and hand inspecting the beans for color and quality.

Traditionally, coffee is a shade-grown plant. It also maintains a high cash value, second only to oil in the international market. Consequently, coffee has helped to preserve rainforest and ecological diversity, unlike beef production and the lumber industry, which have slashed and burned precious forest. Unfortunately, nearly half the world's coffee producers have succumbed to technological advancements and are now producing sun-grown coffee to reap rapid yields and short-term economic gain. These mass-production advantages, however, exact an enormous toll. Sun-grown coffee requires heavier chemical inputs, is more costly to maintain, and drastically depletes the lifespan of the plant. It also has transformed coffee plantations into ecological deserts where fauna and flora are unable to survive, and land degradation, water pollution, and chemical poisoning are rampant. In addition, sun-grown coffee has decimated indigenous cultures who encounter ongoing health hazards and face economic devastation.

Coffee, like tea and cocoa, contains caffeine, a stimulant that affects many parts of the body including the nervous system, kidneys, heart, and gastric system. Caffeine can also be addictive. Decaffeinated coffee has had the caffeine removed by one of two methods before the beans are roasted. The first method is to chemically extract the caffeine with the use of a solvent. The solvent is washed out before the beans are dried, and the roasting process dissolves any remaining residues. The second method, called the Swiss water process, involves steaming the beans and then scraping away the caffeine-rich outer layers.

Some people believe that caffeine is harmful to our health. Others claim that the methods employed in growing coffee are unsound and unjust. From these perspectives, one could question whether coffee is indeed a vegan product. Certainly, the use of coffee is not one of the most exigent issues confronting vegans, and many might contend that what they do to their own bodies is solely their own business. Nevertheless, if coffee-drinking vegans are concerned about the humaneness, environmental soundness, or healthfulness of coffee—as is appropriate for anyone attempting to live a fully compassionate life—they can eliminate it or use it in moderation and seek out only sustainably produced shade-grown coffee that is marketed in accordance with internationally recognized fair trade standards. Organic, shade-grown coffee can usually be found in food cooperatives, natural food stores, and some specialty coffee shops. If it is not labeled as such, be sure to inquire.

Planning Nutritious Meals

I need some school lunch ideas for my vegan children that won't make them stand out from the other kids.

Many foods that are common fare for children are naturally vegan, such as peanut butter and jelly sandwiches or noodles with tomato sauce. There are also numerous instant, frozen, and ready-to-eat prepared foods available in natural food stores that correspond to their nonvegan counterparts, including vegan burgers, tofu dogs, and luncheon "meats." Homemade vegetable pizza can be made easily with English muffins or French bread, jarred sauce, and vegan Parmesan cheese substitute and warmed up in the microwave or toaster oven or packed cold.

Kids of all ages love finger foods. Try packing baked corn chips with salsa, pretzels, boxed cereal, trail mix, crackers or rice cakes with nut butter, dried fruit, raw or dry-roasted nuts, fresh berries, sliced fruit, or vegetable sticks. These all make healthful treats that won't seem peculiar. Smoothies made with fresh or frozen fruit and fortified soy, nut, or grain milk are satisfying and delicious and can be kept cold in a beverage thermos. If you don't have time to make something yourself, pick up some packaged vegan shakes, fruit drinks, and puddings at the natural food store. These handy goodies are great for any age, have a lengthy shelf life, and make a welcome lunchbox addition.

Many foods that are common fare for children are naturally vegan.

Keep frozen vegetable pizzas, burritos, and vegan stuffed pockets on hand at home. They can be heated up in the evening, then refrigerated and taken cold for lunch. Instant and canned soups can be heated at home and packed in a wide-mouth thermos designed for that purpose. You can also pack noodles (with a little olive oil and nutritional yeast flakes, chunked tomatoes or tomato sauce, or a creamy uncheese sauce) or precooked vegan hot dogs in the same kind of thermos. Vegan muffins are convenient and tasty and make a satisfying accompaniment to soup or salad.

Try preparing bean dips, such as hummus, or tofu eggless spreads for high-protein sandwich fillers. Stuff them into pita pockets or pack along crackers for an interesting switch from bread. Some children even like plain lettuce and tomato sandwiches with just a little vegan mayonnaise or bagels with jelly or vegan cream cheese.

It's easy to find conventional foods that are vegan as well as tasty vegan analogs, and it's not hard to adapt vegan foods to individual tastes. With the vast array of prepared products available, there's bound to be a slew of options your children will like. Many large supermarkets now carry some organic produce, soy milk, tofu, veggie burgers, and other prepared vegan foods. You may have to explore the shelves and read a few labels, but there's a good chance you'll find a number of vegan products right in your mainstream store.

If you're lucky enough to have a natural food store near you, it's well worth taking a trip there. Even smaller independent stores and midsize retail establishments offer a good selection of fresh organic produce along with all kinds of great prepared vegan foods. You're certain to find plenty to stock up with.

If there's a vegetarian society in your area, consider joining or going to a meeting. Get-togethers and share-a-dish meals are great ways to get ideas from other parents and swap recipes. And don't forget to talk to your kids directly to find out what they would most prefer. Sometimes the simplest solutions are as close as the nearest hug. When children feel their input is valued and respected, they'll be glad to offer their suggestions–especially regarding matters of the stomach.

I am in high school and have been a vegetarian for over half of my life. I really want to become a vegan but I feel that it would be hard since I am such an active person. For instance, what can I eat at lunchtime at school that will fill me up but is not a slice of pizza or a candy bar?

For most young vegans, unless they live in an exceptionally vegan-friendly town, it is much easier to fix something at home to eat than it is to find something edible and satisfying in the school cafeteria. Even though you may feel rushed in the morning, it is important that you eat a well-balanced breakfast. A nutritious morning meal that fills you up can go a long way toward boosting your energy and getting you through the day.

Whenever possible, pack a lunch for yourself. Sandwiches are always quick and easy. You can try bean spread, nut butter and jelly, vegan cheese, baked or smoked tofu, or seitan-based luncheon meat. (Seitan is a chewy, succulent, meatlike product made from gluten, the protein in wheat.) Before or after dinner, cook frozen prepared veggie burgers, hot dogs, vegetable pockets, or burritos to bring for lunch the following day. Carry a thermos of boiled water and a packet of instant soup or a meal-in-a-cup and prepare it just before lunchtime. Alternatively, before school in the morning, heat up leftover or canned soup, baked beans, or spaghetti with tomato sauce and pack it into a wide-mouth thermos designed specifically for hot foods. Vegan hot dogs can also be kept hot when stored in boiling water in a wide-mouth thermos. Make or buy a bean dip (such as hummus) and bring pita bread and some vegetable sticks. Small boxes of cold cereal along with soy milk in aseptic packages and fresh fruit make a simple, easy-to-pack lunch. If you have time after school or on the weekend, make a big batch of soup, pasta salad, or rice salad to use throughout the week.

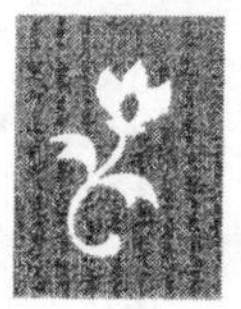

For most young vegans it is much easier to fix something at home to eat than it is to find something edible in the school cafeteria.

Keep a stash of ready-to-eat foods in your backpack: fresh and dried fruit (such as raisins, apricots, and fruit leather), fruit juice in small bottles or aseptic packages, soy milk or rice milk in aseptic packages, vegan pudding cups, granola, trail mix, soy nuts, plain popcorn, pretzels, baked corn chips, crackers (plain or spread with nut butter), and vegan sports bars. If there is a natural food store near you, take the time to look over the shelves to find new and exciting portable foods. Don't forget to look in the deli case and freezer section, too. There are many prepared foods that travel well and frozen items that you could heat up at home in the evening and take to school cold the next day. Some natural food stores even have their own bakery and may offer vegan cookies and muffins.

Being vegan is not vastly different from being vegetarian. You are already most of the way there. With just a little extra planning, you should have no difficulty making the change. And, once you do, no matter how hectic your life is, being vegan will eventually become comfortable and effortless. After a while it will no longer be a process—it will simply be an integral part of who you are.

My niece, who lives with me, is vegan, and I am trying to convince her to cook something other than beans and rice. The rest of my family is not vegan—in fact, not even vegetarian—so I need recipes that can win them over occasionally. I find purchasing prepared products to be quite expensive. Any suggestions?

Beans and whole grains are nourishing, low-fat, high-fiber foods, which are staples for myriad cultures around the world. They also form the foundation of many vegetarian diets. There are innumerable varieties of both beans and grains, so not only are they healthful, wholesome, and inexpensive, they are exciting. Nevertheless, many people who are current or former meat-eaters aren't enamored by a regimen of strictly beans and grains. And, of course, for a well-rounded vegan diet, one must also include plenty of fresh vegetables, fruits, nuts, and seeds.

There is a vast array of packaged and prepared vegan foods available in natural food stores and many supermarkets. These are usually quite delicious, and there are enough different manufacturers that if you don't like one company's products you can always try another's. You're right, however, that a diet centered around these items could become very pricey.

Vegan cooking doesn't have to be fancy, exotic, or costly. A simple baked potato with a little olive oil or low-fat salad dressing, steamed vegetables, and a salad can make a satisfying and economical dinner. Other familiar options are pasta with tomato sauce, stir-fried vegetables with rice, or black bean chili with cracked wheat and vegetables. Tortillas filled with mashed and seasoned pinto beans, lettuce, tomato, onions, olives, salsa and avocado is yet another quick and tasty meal. Many common foods like these are so familiar that people sometimes forget they're eating vegetarian.

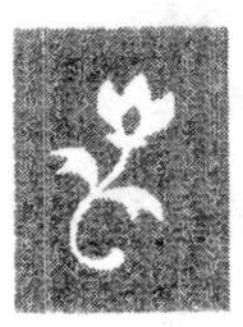

Vegan cooking doesn't have to be fancy, exotic, or costly.

What's particularly enjoyable about being vegan is that there are no strict rules for how to plan a meal. You can certainly eat in the style of the standard American diet if you want to–veggie burgers on whole wheat buns with all the trimmings, tofu hot dogs, cereal with soymilk, nondairy ice cream, meat analogs, vegetable-topped pizza, and so forth. But vegan diets open the door to many new and exhilarating ideas. You can use your imagination to conjure up any combination of foods that sounds appealing and no one will tell you "That's not allowed!" Compared to what most North Americans regularly consume, the vegan diet inspires continual creativity and offers an incredible amount of joy and freedom.

I'm really interested in getting started with a totally vegetarian diet. Because of my hurried schedule I usually try to buy quick-fix meals, but I find that most are too spicy and I don't like them. What can I do?

The search for prepared foods that suit your individual tastes requires an investment of time and money. There is simply no short-cut solution. You've got to buy the product to determine whether or not you like it. It's a gamble, of course, because you run the risk of purchasing something that neither you nor anyone else in your household will eat. Occasionally, natural food stores provide free tastings of products they carry, often in conjunction with a special promotion. These are great opportunities to sample products without any financial outlay. Try to find out when these events are scheduled so you can be sure to attend. If there is something in particular you've been wanting to try, ask the manager if samples of this item could be available at the same time. Retailers want to please their customers, so it's always worth inquiring.

The only foolproof way to ensure that a dish will please your palate is to make it yourself. Even with a hectic lifestyle, it's still possible to prepare healthful foods from scratch at home. Mainly it requires organization and forethought. But even for longer-cooking foods, such as beans and grains, the effort is relatively minimal. Beans can be soaked overnight or during the day while you are at work. Alternatively, they can be quick-soaked in boiling water. Cover rinsed beans with water, bring to a boil, then put a lid on the pot and set the beans aside to rest for an hour. If you pressure-cook your beans, they can be ready in minutes instead of hours. Grains can also be pressure-cooked, although this method just minimally reduces the overall cooking time. Even with stovetop simmering, though, grains require very little tending. You can start them cooking as soon as you get home, then go about unwinding or preparing the rest of your meal, and before you know it they'll be ready. It helps to cook large batches of longer-cooking foods and store them in the refrigerator to use throughout the week. Cooked beans and grains are ideal to use in salads, add to soups, or simply reheat (leftover grains are best steamed or stir-fried) and season to your taste.

Lettuce, fresh vegetables, and fruits can be washed in the evening, over the weekend, or whenever you have time off. Pat them dry and store them in the refrigerator packed in breathable and reusable storage bags designed specifically for this purpose or wrapped in a clean tea towel. Having ready-to-use produce on hand will speed up meal preparation enormously.

Fixing home-cooked dishes allows you to regulate all the ingredients so that you are assured of the most healthful meals. As a bonus, when you make recipes from scratch, *you* control the seasonings instead of a manufacturer.

My college dining hall doesn't offer much in the way of vegan food, so I end up eating mostly side dishes. I try to do a little cooking in my dorm room, but this isn't always possible. I'm concerned about getting enough to eat. Any ideas?

Depending on what is offered, the side dishes from the dining hall could make up a reasonably healthful meal. However, you are right to be concerned about getting adequate nutrition. If balanced meals are not available on campus, you will need to use a little creativity.

As long as you have access to a refrigerator, regardless of how small, a burner, a pot or two, and maybe a microwave or toaster oven, you should be able to cook up a few dishes or heat up a few packaged or prepared foods. Here are some ideas to spark your imagination:

> *Breakfast:* soy yogurt, bagels, toast, cold cereal, instant oatmeal, other instant hot cereal grains, fresh fruit
>
> *Lunch or dinner:* sandwich of peanut butter and jelly or lettuce, bean spread with crackers or bread, canned or instant soup (particularly convenient if the dining hall has hot water available for tea or other hot beverages), noodles with tomato sauce (easy to heat up in your room), veggie burger or vegan hot dog on a bun, cold pasta or vegetable salad, instant mashed potatoes, canned or instant chili, whole wheat tortilla stuffed with veggies from the dining hall salad bar
>
> *Snacks:* fresh and dried fruit, trail mix, dry cereal, granola, vegan sports bars, pretzels, baked corn chips with salsa, crackers with nut butter, juices and nondairy milks in aseptic packages

If you have access to a natural food store or well-stocked supermarket, you may find handy prepared items such as spinach pies, vegan burritos, bean dips, and salads. If there is a fast-food restaurant near campus, you could order a plain baked potato or make one in your room or apartment. They're surprisingly good with just ketchup and can be very filling when topped with a thick bean soup or spread, vegetarian canned baked beans, or tofu sour cream. Most natural food stores have lots of portable vegan desserts such as sweet muffins, cookies, and pudding cups, as well as frozen nondairy desserts. These can often be costly, however, and are frequently not the most wholesome choices.

If you have access to an oven, you could occasionally host a dinner party with a few friends and make some special vegan meals and treats to share. If enough students and faculty are interested, you might even want to talk to the food service director or circulate a petition on campus to have vegan meals served regularly in the dining hall.

I am sixteen and currently a vegetarian but aspire to be a vegan, I just don't know how to go about it in a healthy fashion. I still live with my parents and they shop for groceries. They have accepted me being a vegetarian, but they are reluctant to support me in being vegan. Can you help me compile a shopping list of foods and direct me to some excellent recipes?

It is wonderful that your parents have supported you in your choice to be vegetarian, since a lot of young people are not as fortunate. Your parents are probably concerned about your desire to switch to veganism because they, like you, want to make sure you maintain a healthful diet. In addition, since it appears they are responsible for the bulk of grocery shopping and food preparation, they may feel pressured to learn about new foods and recipes. The more you are willing to help relieve them of these extra burdens, the more likely it is that they will accept your decision to become vegan.

Even though your parents shop and pay for the groceries, don't leave your food choices strictly up to them. Since you are the only one in the family who is vegetarian (on her way to becoming vegan), and you are essentially the only person who will be eating these foods, it should be your responsibility to determine what you need and want them to buy for you. Learn as much as you can about proper vegan nutrition so you can make wise choices.

Visit your local bookstore and browse through the vegan cookbooks. Pick one or two with recipes that sound easy and appealing. Don't be put off by a few ingredients that seem unusual. Most vegan recipe books have glossaries that explain what these ingredients are and how to use them. A trip to a natural food store once or twice a month should be sufficient to supply you with any new foods you may want to try. Most large grocery stores carry an array of vegan specialty items such as nondairy milk, regular and silken tofu, and frozen, packaged, and prepared foods, which, although more expensive than cooking from scratch, can make fixing meals a breeze on hectic days. Vegan staples such as fruits, vegetables, beans, grains, nuts, seeds, pasta, potatoes, pita bread, tortillas, and cheeseless pizza shells are readily available everywhere.

The more you know about how to devise a healthful vegan diet, the easier it will be to map out a meal chart based on nutritious recipes and snacks you know you will like. Work with seven days at a time (three meals a day plus snacks) to plan for five weekdays and one weekend. From there you can create a weekly grocery list for the ingredients and foods you will need. Give the list to your parents, or better yet, offer to go to the store with them or on your own. And don't wait for one of the adults to make the recipes for you. Offer to prepare them yourself, and to clean up afterward, too. You may even want to propose cooking a vegan dish for the whole family on occasion. It could be fun for everyone and would be a nice break for your parents, which might make them all the more receptive to your veganism.

If you believe you are mature enough to make the decision to be vegan, prove it to yourself and to your family by demonstrating initiative and responsibility. You'll feel more independent, and your parents will be impressed with your motivation, thoughtfulness, and obvious commitment to your ideals.

I live in a very cold region where nine months out of the year snow covers the ground and fruits and vegetables are hard to come by. I'm a picky eater to begin with. How would you recommend I go about becoming vegan?

Rest assured that there are vegans throughout the world, including others just like you in frigid and remote places. With commitment and perhaps a little ingenuity, it's possible to be vegan practically anywhere. Your only hurdle is being a picky eater, which would make obtaining good nutrition a challenge whether or not you were vegan.

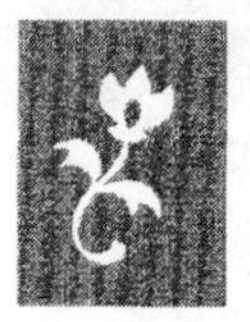

With commitment and a little ingenuity,
it's possible to be vegan practically anywhere.

Fresh fruits and vegetables are available in virtually all mainstream supermarkets, regardless of where you live. Although they may not be locally or organically grown, they are certainly the next best thing. If you are unable to obtain fresh produce, you should still have ready access to frozen fruits and vegetables and, in a pinch, canned ones. The question is, will you eat them?

In addition to vegetables and fruits, a well-planned vegan diet should incorporate a wide variety of foods including whole grains, legumes, nuts, and seeds. Many stores and supermarkets carry frozen veggie burgers and meat analogs as well as seasoned vegetable combinations that merely require the addition of tofu or beans to make a quick and complete main dish. If you don't have a natural food store near you, a number of mail-order sources ship nonperishable vegan foods such as soups and quick mixes for everything from seitan to burgers to dips to brownies.

Don't overlook the simple standards that even most nonvegans enjoy, such as pasta with marinara or mushroom sauce, baked potatoes with broccoli and tofu sour cream or a nondairy cheese sauce, or bean burritos with all the trimmings. Ethnic cuisine offers lots of excitement and variety, so be sure to consider these specialties as well.

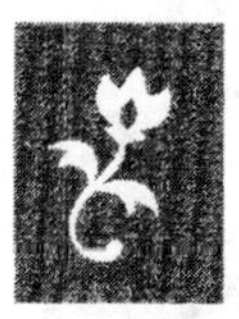

Once people become comfortable with the idea
of being vegan, they typically find more culinary
delights than they ever expected.

Indulge in one or two vegan cookbooks that have recipes incorporating the foods and flavors you most prefer. Spend a few hours a week experimenting in the kitchen just to have fun trying out some new dishes. Vegan living, as well as vegan eating, is really a series of discoveries. Once people become comfortable with the idea of being vegan, they typically find more culinary delights than they ever expected.

Don't box yourself in or feel you must eat certain foods. If you are extremely particular about what you will and won't eat, it is especially important to read up on vegan nutrition. If you are concerned that you are not obtaining sufficient nutrients because you are avoiding entire categories of foods, then by all means consult with a nutritionist or dietitian who is familiar with vegan diets.

I was recently on a school trip. We stopped off at a fast-food chain to eat dinner. Being a vegan, I would never think about eating at a place like this, but since I had no other choice, I ordered a salad. Is it wrong for a vegan to buy or endorse anything from a fast-food corporation that primarily sells hamburgers?

Vegans are mixed about going to fast-food restaurants. Most tend to avoid them because they have so little, and often nothing, for vegans to eat. In addition, fast foods that may appear vegan-friendly frequently contain animal products. For instance, some franchises prefry their french fries in beef fat. Gelatin is a common thickening agent used in fast-food salad dressings. Buns often contain whey, refried beans and wraps may contain lard, and pizza sauce and crusts often contain cheese or other dairy products. Complicating matters further, there is sometimes no consistency from region to region. For example, a restaurant chain in the Northeast may offer a vegan pasta sauce, but the sauce in the Midwest may contain beef broth.

Then there is the issue of having one's money support a business that deals almost exclusively in animal products. Vegans are torn on this matter as well. For some vegans, fast food is a great help to them when they travel or are in a rush and there is nothing else available. Many vegans would be thrilled to be able to go to a totally vegan franchise where there would be excellent options and no conflict of conscience. On the other hand, some vegans feel that if they purchase the few vegan offerings that a burger chain provides, they are voting for the company to continue to carry these items (or expand their vegetarian line) and also letting them know they are not supporting their animal products.

If you are in a bind (such as your school trip), there may be no option. Many vegans who travel have no choice but to occasionally get a salad or baked potato at a burger stop. When you're hungry and there is nothing else around, it's certainly a reasonable alternative. As a steady diet, it may not be the best vegan way to invest your money. Nevertheless, as a short-term interim solution, it is sometimes the best deal going.

Working with Staples

Is it necessary to steam tofu before using it? Will the consistency change with steaming?

Regular tofu, also known as Chinese tofu, is commonly sold in bulk or individual tubs, refrigerated and packed in water. After opening, the tofu should be submerged in water and kept in an airtight container in the refrigerator. The water should be drained off daily. Then the tofu should be rinsed and covered again with fresh water.

Because tofu is a moist, high-protein food, bacteria on it will grow rapidly. Unlike some brands of silken tofu that are packaged in aseptic boxes, fresh tofu is not hermetically sealed. Therefore, as a precaution, water-packed tofu should be simmered in water or steamed for five to ten minutes before using in uncooked recipes, such as tofu salad. Most recipes do not specify this extra step, but from a safety angle it is definitely worth doing.

Many cooks find simmering or steaming water-packed tofu to be advantageous for another reason as well. After the tofu has cooked briefly and cooled, it becomes firmer. For most dishes, this firmer product works beautifully and enhances the texture of the finished recipe.

Be sure to cool steamed or simmered tofu quickly and thoroughly before using it in uncooked recipes. The best method is to cut it into half-inch to one-inch-thick slices and place it in a single layer in a shallow metal, glass, or ceramic pan. Place the pan on a cooling rack in the refrigerator and let the tofu chill, uncovered, until all the pieces feel cold. Occasionally turn the pieces over and rearrange them, because the ones around the edge of the pan will cool more quickly than those in the center.

Is TVP vegan? If so, how do I use it?

The initials *TVP* stand for textured vegetable protein, a food product made from soybeans. It has been manufactured for over twenty years by the Archer Daniels Midland Company of Decatur, Illinois. TVP is produced from defatted soy flour that is cooked under pressure and extruded into flakes, granules, or chunks.

TVP flakes and granules provide a texture similar to ground beef and are an excellent replacement in conventional recipes that typically contain meat, such as chili, tacos, sloppy joes, and spaghetti sauce. TVP chunks can be used to replace meat strips in stews or stir-fries. They are also available flavored to taste like ham, beef, or chicken.

Dry TVP must be rehydrated and cooked. One cup of TVP flakes or granules rehydrated in ⅞ cup of boiling water will provide 2 cups of hydrated TVP for use in your favorite recipes. The larger chunks must be covered with water and simmered for several minutes. Because TVP is a dry product with a very low fat content, it has a long shelf life and will keep indefinitely. Store it in airtight containers to keep out moisture. All TVP, plain or flavored, is vegan.

Is there any *simple* way to cook brown rice—a good rule of thumb? I can't seem to make it consistently, and I usually burn it. I need a good basic rice recipe.

Like many whole grains, brown rice takes a while to cook, but the process is virtually effortless. For *most* whole grains (but not all), the standard rule of thumb is about 2 cups water to 1 cup grain. This is a good guide for brown rice, too, although short-grain brown rice requires slightly more water than long grain.

Here is a reliable standard recipe for brown rice. The oil is optional, although it makes for a more tender rice. It is essential that you turn the burner to the absolute lowest setting after the water comes to a boil *and* that you use a pot with a very tight-fitting lid. Otherwise, steam will escape and the rice will have a greater tendency to burn. If the heat on your burner cannot go down very low, slip a flame tamer under the pot. This will also help to keep the rice from scorching. For long-grain brown rice, use a scant 2 cups of water. For short-grain brown rice, it's a good idea to add an extra ¼ to ½ cup of water, especially if you like your rice soft rather than dry and fluffy, or if the lid of your pot is not snug.

Check the rice after 45 to 50 minutes. Spread the grains apart with a fork, and if there is still water in the bottom of the pot, put the lid back on and continue to let it cook for 10 to 15 minutes longer. If there is no water in the bottom of the pot, and the rice is making a sizzling sound, the rice is finished cooking. Remove it from the heat at once and continue with step 2 of the directions.

PERFECTLY COOKED BROWN RICE

Makes about 3 servings.

2 to 2½ cups filtered water
1 cup brown rice (rinsed well in a mesh colander and drained)
1 tablespoon canola or olive oil (optional)
½ teaspoon salt

1. Place the water, rice, oil, and salt in a heavy saucepan. Bring to a boil. Immediately reduce the heat to very low and cover the pot with a tight-fitting lid. Cook undisturbed for 45 to 50 minutes. (Do not stir the rice or peek inside the pot until the end of the cooking time!)
2. Fluff with a fork so the drier grains are on top. Place a clean tea towel over the pot. Replace the lid snugly (over the towel) and let rest for 5 to 10 minutes. (The towel will absorb excess moisture.) Fluff again and serve.

Is the peel of washed fruit or vegetables harmful to us?

The peels of certain fruits and vegetables are extremely thick, tough, or bad tasting, making them difficult if not impossible to chew and digest.

For example, avocado skin, melon rind, banana peels,.and corn husks are simply not edible. The skins of many other plant foods, however, are not only tender and delicious but are often considered the most nutritious part. With many fruits and vegetables, the richest source of nutrients lies just below the skin. When this part is removed and discarded, along with it go not only valuable nutrients but important dietary fiber.

On the other hand, pesticides and herbicides are most concentrated on the surface of fruits and vegetables, and frequently they are absorbed much more deeply. From a health perspective, it is never smart to consume toxic chemicals. Therefore, if your fruits and vegetables are grown conventionally, it is wise to make a habit of peeling most produce.

Even if your food is organically produced, all fruits and vegetables should be thoroughly cleaned before consumption. Most soil harbors dangerous bacteria and other microorganisms that can be harmful to your health if ingested. In addition, a large number of commercially grown produce is also waxed. Waxes repel water, provide a protective coating, and create a glossy finish for greater visual appeal. Food-grade waxes may be vegetable, synthetic, or animal derived. Shellac, which is made from lac, a resinous substance secreted by the female lac insect, is commonly used in combination with food-grade waxes. Fruit and vegetable washes and sprays designed specifically for removing chemical residue, wax, dirt, and bacteria are readily available in supermarkets and natural food stores. Alternatively, you could use warm soapy water along with a vegetable brush or clean dishcloth. Washing is an important part of food preparation, especially if you do not peel your produce.

Some of the recipes in my cookbooks call for soymilk and others call for nondairy milk. Is there a difference? Can I use rice milk or nut milk instead of soymilk, or is one or the other better for cooking or baking?

Soymilk is an all-purpose plant milk that can be used in cooking as well as baking. It also is a good choice for cream-style soups and sauces. Soymilk is generally less sweet than rice milk or nut milk, which adds to its versatility. Rice milk and nut milk are excellent for use in most baked goods. Whether or not you like them in savory cooked foods, however, is a matter of personal preference. Rice milk is typically thinner and more watery than either soymilk or nut milk.

Regardless of which milk you select, be sure that it is plain, that is, no vanilla, carob, chocolate, or almond flavoring, unless, of course, the recipe specifies a flavor. Most vegan cookbooks just state soymilk when referring to the general category of nondairy milks. If you do not want to use soy, you can substitute rice milk, nut milk, oat milk, mixed grain milk, or other nondairy milks that are available at natural food stores. The taste may vary slightly from what the recipe developer intended, but with the majority of recipes you shouldn't be able to tell the difference.

The Vegan Sweet Tooth

I am trying to figure out why some vegans don't eat plain old sugar that you buy at the grocery store. Can you please explain?

Half of the white table sugar manufactured in the United States is cane sugar and the other half is beet sugar. The primary distinction between the two, other than being derived from different plants, is the processing method. Unlike beet sugar, cane sugar processing typically takes place at two locations, the sugar mill and the refinery. During the final purification process, cane sugar is filtered through activated carbon (charcoal), which may be of animal, vegetable, or mineral origin. This step is unnecessary for beet sugar and therefore is never done.

Approximately half of the cane refineries in the United States use bone char (charcoal made from animal bones) as their activated carbon source. The bone char used in this filtering process is so far removed from its animal source that cane sugar processed in this method is deemed kosher parve, which, according to Jewish dietary laws, means that it contains no meat or milk in any form as an ingredient. There are some vegans who disagree with this perspective, even though bone char does not become part of the final product. Nonetheless, other vegans believe that worrying about bone char processing is pointless.

They consider it a trivial concern that detracts from the primary purpose of vegan living and causes numerous conventional foods that are otherwise vegan to be off limits.

Some vegans replace white table sugar with unbleached cane sugar (often marketed as turbinado or raw sugar) or dehydrated and granulated cane juice, both of which are exempt from bone char filtration. These products can replace white sugar measure for measure for general use and in recipes. However, they are typically darker in color than white table sugar–ranging from light amber to rich brown–due to their naturally higher molasses content. This can sometimes alter the flavor of recipes and may also affect the color of the finished product.

Unbleached cane sugar and dehydrated and granulated cane juice are considered by some to be more healthful than white table sugar. Although they may contain minimal trace nutrients, one would have to eat massive quantities to obtain any dubious nutritive value. And, of course, there are numerous drawbacks associated with the overconsumption of sugar, including tooth decay and obesity.

Beyond the bone char concerns and health-related issues, there are other factors to consider when purchasing sugar and products that contain large quantities of it. The vast majority of sugarcane is not organically grown, and most sugar plantations employ environmentally unsound agricultural methods, such as heavy insecticide and pesticide use and crop burning, which have a negative impact on soil, air, water, and the health of the workers. Sugarcane production is labor and energy intensive and utilizes large amounts of fossil fuels in processing, filtration, packaging, and transport. Plantation owners typically pay meager wages and provide no benefits, and workers are forced to endure brutal, substandard conditions.

There are a number of reasons why some vegans continue to eat white table sugar while others try to avoid it, why some purchase only organically grown unbleached sugar, and why still others eschew sugar products altogether. A prudent approach may be to reduce our use of all types of sugar, including sugary processed foods, and to train our taste buds to more fully appreciate the natural sweetness of fresh and dried fruits, grain sweeteners, and other whole foods. Still another option is to purchase granulated natural sweeteners such as maple sugar, granular fruit sweetener, and date sugar, or to use natural liquid sweeteners such as pure maple syrup, malt syrup, brown rice syrup, and mixed fruit juice concentrates. These products are available in natural food stores and many supermarkets.

Are brown sugar and powdered sugar vegan?

Brown sugar is white sugar combined with molasses, which gives it a soft texture. Powdered sugar, also called confectioners' sugar, is granulated sugar that has been crushed into a fine powder. Brown sugar and powdered sugar can be made from either sugarcane or sugar beets.

Bone char filtration is used for roughly half the cane sugar produced in the United States. This means that some cane sugar may be purified through charcoal made from animal bones. (Bone residue does *not* become part of the finished product.) There is a split among vegans about whether cane sugar refined with bone char is vegan, and, if not, whether this warrants avoiding all products containing white sugar, since it is virtually impossible for consumers to determine the type of sugar (beet or cane) or the processing methods used.

If we assume that animal-free purity is the criterion for ascertaining whether or not something is vegan, are there any truly vegan foods? In the commercial arena, probably not. Regardless of how they are grown, processed, packed, or freighted, most foods eventually come in contact with animal products, directly or indirectly. So where should vegans draw the line? The most practical approach is the following: If a plant-based food contains no overt animal products or by-products, it is vegan.

From an ethical standpoint, this is the most realistic and constructive way to view not only food but other commodities as well. Modern methods of processing and transporting are so pervasively tainted with animal components that it is counterproductive and ultimately futile for vegans to be concerned about technicalities. In addition, preoccupation with minutia detracts from the more pivotal and purposeful aspects of being vegan.

It is vital that vegans continue to discuss matters of ethical practice. However, it is equally significant to channel energies into those areas of vegan living that are consequential. If vegans avoid products because they disapprove of certain processing methods, no vegans could ride in a car, drink tap water, live in a house, or wear manufactured clothing.

Vegans as individuals must decide the extent to which they want to take their beliefs. There are undoubtedly vegans who feel that sugar is not cruelty-free from the angles of health, worker equity, environmental preservation, and processing. For these vegans, all sugar—white, brown, or powdered—is unacceptable. Still, there are others who feel that from every reasonable perspective sugar is vegan and for whom, in terms of the larger picture, the issue is moot.

As far as I know, molasses is a by-product of cane sugar. Does this mean it isn't vegan?

One step in the refining process of sugarcane and sugar beets involves boiling the juice that is obtained from these plants. This results in a viscous mixture from which sugar crystals are extracted. The remaining dark syrup is called molasses.

Light molasses comes from the first boiling of the sugar syrup. It is pale in color, delicate in flavor, and is the sweetest of the various grades of molasses, making it a good choice to use on pancakes and waffles. Dark molasses comes from a second boiling and is golden brown, thicker, and less sweet than light molasses. It is used mostly in cooking and baking. Blackstrap molasses comes from a third boiling. It is brownish-black, very thick, and somewhat bitter. Blackstrap molasses is a rich source of iron and calcium. Sorghum molasses is the syrup produced from the cereal grain sorghum.

The primary reason that cane sugar may be considered nonvegan by some vegans is because of the possibility that it was filtered through bone char. However, molasses that is obtained from sugarcane is procured long before the sugar crystals are cleaned and filtered. Therefore, all molasses (cane, beet, and sorghum) is vegan.

I know that vegans do not consume honey, but how about other syrups? Are they suitable for a vegan?

You are correct that vegans do not consume honey. Avoiding honey was part of the original 1944 manifesto of The Vegan Society in

England and has always been the position of the American Vegan Society since its founding in 1960. Fortunately, there are many other syrups that vegans can use instead. Here are some of these options:

- *Agave nectar:* A natural liquid sweetener made from the core of the blue agave, a cactus-like plant native to Mexico, best known for its use in making tequila. It has a 93 percent fruit sugar content and is about 25 percent sweeter than sugar. Agave nectar dissolves easily and has a smooth, mild taste.
- *Brown rice syrup:* A subtle sweetener made by combining cooked brown rice with dried sprouted barley and culturing the mixture until malt enzymes convert some of the rice starch into glucose and maltose.
- *Concentrated fruit juice syrups:* Fruit juice that has been refined to remove fiber and impurities and boiled into a syrup.
- *Corn syrup:* An inexpensive, thick syrup made from chemically refined cornstarch.
- *Frozen fruit juice concentrates:* Fruit juice that has been refined to remove fiber and impurities along with approximately two-thirds of the water content.
- *FruitSource (liquid):* A brand-name product made from grape juice concentrate and whole rice syrup, with a taste and consistency similar to honey. Also available granulated.
- *Malt syrup:* A thick, sticky sweetener extracted from roasted, sprouted whole barley, rye, or wheat. It has a light molasses flavor and is about half as sweet as white sugar.
- *Maple syrup:* A highly flavorful and concentrated sweetener; it takes about thirty to forty gallons of sap to produce one gallon of syrup. Be sure to purchase only pure maple syrup. "Maple-flavored syrup" consists primarily of sugar or corn syrup and usually contains artificial coloring and flavoring.

  At one time, maple syrup producers routinely added a small amount of lard, an animal fat, during processing to minimize foaming. In recent years, this practice has been eliminated by nearly all maple syrup companies. Instead, a small quantity of vegetable oil is typically used. If you have a concern and want to verify how your maple syrup was made, contact the producer directly. You can also check the label for a kosher marking. Kosher maple syrup is not processed with lard.

- *Molasses:* The thick, dark syrup that remains after sugar crystals are removed during cane sugar refinement.
- *Sorghum syrup:* A sweet, golden syrup made from the stalks of sorghum, a cereal grain related to millet.

Most natural food stores carry these as well as other alternative sweeteners. It's a good idea to experiment with them to see which ones have the flavors you most prefer. If possible, invest initially in small quantities of several different sweeteners and try them in various recipes before purchasing larger amounts.

Here are some tips for using alternative liquid sweeteners:

- To replace white sugar with a liquid sweetener, reduce the total amount of other liquid ingredients in the recipe by about ¼ cup for each cup of liquid sweetener used.
- To liquify liquid sweetener that has crystallized, place the jar in a pan of hot water for several minutes.
- To accurately measure liquid sweetener and keep it from sticking to the measuring utensil, first rub some oil in your measuring cup or spoon or warm the sweetener in hot water as directed above.

Baking Challenges

What is the difference between whole-wheat, whole-wheat pastry, white-wheat, all-purpose, bread, and pastry flours? Are all of them vegan, and are they interchangeable in recipes?

Whole-wheat flour contains the bran (the fibrous outer layer) and the germ (the part that sprouts) of the whole-wheat berry. Therefore it has a higher nutritional, fiber, and fat profile than white flours, which have had both the bran and germ removed, and whole-wheat flour should be stored in the refrigerator or freezer to prevent rancidity. The texture of whole-wheat flour can range from soft and powdery to coarse, depending on the amount of bolting (sifting) it receives at the mill. Bolting removes some of the coarse bran, making the flour finer.

Bleached white flours not only have had the bran and germ removed, taking with it essential vitamins and nutrients, they have been whitened. White flour can be bleached naturally as it ages, or it can be bleached chemically. Potassium bromate, a chemical used as an oxidizing agent and also used to enhance baking characteristics, has been added regularly to some white flours for a long time. Potassium bromate has been banned in Europe, Japan, and Canada. In California, flours containing this chemical must carry a label warning of its potential as a carcinogen. Unbleached white flours also have had their natural bran and germ removed, but they have not undergone a bleaching process. These flours retain more of the natural warm, golden color of wheat than snowy-white bleached flours. By U.S. law, wheat flours that do not contain the germ must be enriched with niacin, riboflavin, thiamin, and iron, all of which are derived for commercial purposes from vegan sources.

All-purpose flours are a blend of high-gluten hard wheat and low-gluten soft wheat and may be used, as the name implies, for all purposes, from thickening sauces and soups to making pastries and yeast bread. Depending on the recipe, however, some baked goods made with all-purpose flour may provide less than satisfactory results.

Pastry flour (white or whole-wheat) is made from soft winter wheat, which has a higher starch and lower gluten content. Pastry flour produces the finest, most tender pie crusts and pastries, biscuits, muffins, and scones. Whole wheat pastry flour is more nutritious than white flour, but it can make baked goods seem heavy and crumbly. Also, since most conventional pastry recipes call for white flour, when you substitute whole-wheat pastry flour you may discover that you need to adjust the quantity of liquid used. Many people who are accustomed to a refined diet but want to adopt a more wholesome way of eating find that using a mixture of half unbleached white flour (pastry or all-purpose) and half whole-wheat pastry flour in their recipes makes their pastries and nonyeasted baked goods lighter and more palatable than if only whole-wheat flour were used.

White whole-wheat flour is milled from hard white winter wheat, a new and exciting variety that offers a lot of versatility. It does not have the strong flavor and dark color of traditional whole-wheat flour but, since it includes the entire wheat berry, it contains the fiber-rich bran and mineral-rich germ. Substitute white whole-wheat flour for all-purpose or pastry flour in your cookie, muffin, cake, brownie, pancake, and quick-bread recipes, or try it in whole-wheat yeast bread for a lighter-colored, milder-tasting loaf.

Bread flour–white or whole-wheat–is made from high-protein, hard red spring wheat. The extra gluten (protein) in this flour means yeast bread will rise more strongly and vigorously. Do not substitute pastry flour for bread flour in yeast bread recipes. Conversely, do not substitute bread flour for all-purpose or pastry flour in nonyeasted baked goods. Different flours will contain varying amounts of moisture depending on the type of flour, its age, and how it was stored. Therefore, you may need to adjust the amount of liquid needed in your recipes.

Although some flours are more nutritious than others, all flours are vegan.

What can I use instead of eggs in my favorite baked goods, burgers, and loaves? I've tried commercial egg replacers, but the cakes don't rise or the ingredients don't bind.

Eggs are typically used to lighten baked goods or to hold ingredients together. In most recipes that do not require much leavening and call for only one egg, simply omit the egg. However, for recipes that require a large quantity of eggs or egg whites (such as angel food cake or meringue topping), no substitute yet exists that provides a comparable outcome.

Here are several suggestions to lighten and bind baked goods. Each is the equivalent of one medium egg:

- Finely grind 1 tablespoon whole flaxseeds in a dry electric blender or seed mill, or use 2½ tablespoons preground flaxseeds.

(Flaxseeds fluff when they are ground, thus the disparity in the measurement between the whole and ground seeds. Always store ground flaxseeds in the freezer, because they are highly perishable.) Transfer to a bowl and beat in 3 to 4 tablespoons of water using a wire whisk or a fork. This mixture is not only an excellent replacement for eggs, it also contributes healthful lignins (a special fiber that may provide protection against certain diseases) and vital omega-3 fatty acids.

- ¼ cup mashed soft tofu blended with the liquid called for in the recipe.
- ¼ cup mashed banana or applesauce beaten with ½ teaspoon double-acting baking powder.
- 1 heaping tablespoon soy flour or garbanzo bean flour beaten with 1 tablespoon water.
- 2 tablespoons flour, 1½ teaspoons canola oil, and ½ teaspoon double-acting baking powder beaten with 2 tablespoons water.

The rise of cakes usually has more to do with the leavening ingredients than with the eggs. Baking powder is perishable and should be kept in a cool dry place. It also has a shelf life, and its potency will diminish as that date draws near. To test if your baking powder is still viable, mix 1 teaspoon with ⅓ cup hot water. If it does not bubble vigorously, discard it. Most vegan bakers find that double-acting baking powder, which releases gas when it becomes wet and again when it is exposed to oven heat, provides the best results. If your recipe calls for baking soda, you can add a little vinegar to the liquid ingredients to give it some extra punch. About 2 teaspoons for each 8-inch cake or layer should do the trick.

To bind veggie burgers, loaves, and casseroles, mix in one or more of the following, adding just enough to make the mixture the consistency of very thick cooked cereal:

- starch (such as arrowroot powder, kuzu, potato starch, or cornstarch)
- flour (such as oat, soy, garbanzo, whole-wheat, spelt, barley, rye, or rice)

- dry rolled oats or cooked oatmeal
- bread crumbs, cracker meal, or matzo meal
- finely crushed cornflakes
- instant potato flakes
- mashed potatoes
- mashed sweet potatoes
- nut or seed butters
- tomato paste
- nondairy white sauce
- soft tofu blended with a little flour (use 4 parts tofu to 1 part flour)

Veganizing recipes that call for eggs sometimes takes a bit of experimentation. Be sure to write down exactly what you do, so if you like the results, you'll be able to duplicate them the next time you want to make the recipe.

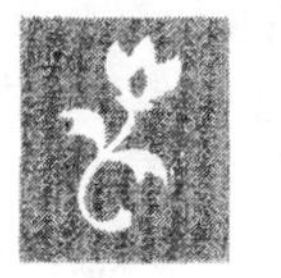

Epilogue

There is a special joy connected with vegan living that is unattainable almost anywhere else. Because there are no conflicts of conscience, an indescribable inner peace coincides with vegan practice. This serenity is the direct corollary of implementing conscious compassion and choosing to employ a lifestyle of ethical consistency. Thus vegans are free to experience empathy for and mutual respect among all life forms because there is no illusory line that separates our spirits. Vegans acknowledge that the life force within people is the same life energy abiding in all living beings. We are identical in that regard; we are kin. The air, water, earth, and sky are shared by all who inhabit this span of time and space. What an awe-inspiring realization!

In recognizing our place within the scheme of existence, vegans can participate in harmony with all creation. There is no need to align ourselves hierarchically if we are part of a united pool of energy. In this light it becomes nonsensical to think in terms that separate us from each other. With this understanding, vegans hold a key to solving our numerous problems personally, locally, nationally, and globally. Veganism is the liberation of spirit and reason, and it is available to everyone everywhere. It is the gift of truthfulness, integrity, justice, respect, love, awareness, and choice. To receive it, you need only open your heart.

Joanne Stepaniak conducts compassionate living workshops and lectures throughout North America. If you would like to arrange a presentation for your group or organization, please contact her at P.O. Box 82663, Swissvale, PA 15218, or visit her Web site, Grassroots Veganism, at www.vegsource.com/joanne.

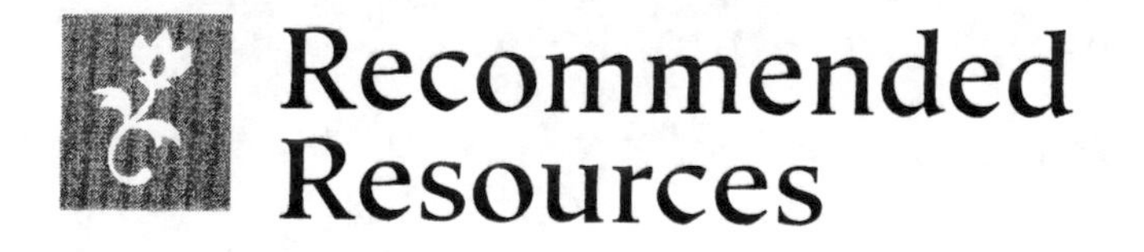

Recommended Resources

Books

Coe, Sue, and Alexander Cockburn. *Dead Meat.* New York: Four Walls Eight Windows, 1996.

Davis, Karen. *Prisoned Chickens, Poisoned Eggs.* Summertown, Tenn.: Book Publishing Company, 1996.

Eisnitz, Gail. *Slaughterhouse: The Shocking Story of Greed, Neglect, and Inhumane Treatment Inside the U.S. Meat Industry.* Buffalo, N.Y.: Prometheus Books, 1997.

Hanh, Tich Nhat. *Peace Is Every Step: The Path to Mindfulness in Everyday Life.* New York: Bantam Books, 1991.

Krizmanic, Judy. *A Teen's Guide to Going Vegetarian.* New York: Puffin, 1994.

Melina, Vesanto, Brenda Davis, and Victoria Harrison. *Becoming Vegetarian.* Summertown, Tenn.: Book Publishing Company, 1995.

Messina, Virginia, and Mark Messina. *The Vegetarian Way.* New York: Crown Trade Paperbacks, 1996.

Peace Pilgrim: Her Life and Work in Her Own Words, compiled by some of her friends. Santa Fe, N.M.: Ocean Tree Books, 1992.

Robbins, John. *Diet for a New America.* Tiburon, Calif.: HJ Kramer, 1989.

Stepaniak, Joanne. *The Vegan Sourcebook,* 2nd ed. Los Angeles: Lowell House, 2000.

Videos, Pamphlets, and Information

The American Anti-Vivisection Society (AAVS), 801 Old York Road, No. 204, Jenkintown, Pennsylvania 19046. Phone: (215) 887-0816. Fax: (215) 887-2088.

The American Vegan Society (AVS), P.O. Box 369, Malaga, New Jersey 08328. Phone: (856) 694-2887. Fax: (856) 694-2288.

EarthSave International, 1509 Seabright Avenue, Suite B1, Santa Cruz, California 95062. Phone: 1-800-362-3648.

Farm Animal Reform Movement (FARM), P.O. Box 30654, Bethesda, Maryland 20824. Phone: (301) 530-1737. Fax: (301) 530-5747.

Farm Sanctuary East, P.O. Box 150, Watkins Glen, New York 14891. Phone: (607) 583-2225.

Farm Sanctuary West, P.O. Box 1065, Orland, California 95963. Phone: (530) 865-4617.

The Fund for Animals, World Building, 8121 Georgia Avenue, Suite 301, Silver Spring, Maryland 20910. Phone: (301) 585-2591. Fax: (301) 585-2595.

Humane Society of the United States (HSUS), 2100 L Street NW, Washington, DC 20037. Phone: (202) 452-1100. Fax: (202) 778-6132.

North American Vegetarian Society (NAVS), P.O. Box 72, Dolgeville, New York 13329. Phone: (518) 568-7970. Fax: (518) 568-7979.

People for the Ethical Treatment of Animals (PETA), 501 Front Street, Norfolk, Virginia 23510. Phone: (757) 622-7382. Fax: (757) 622-0457.

Physicians Committee for Responsible Medicine (PCRM), 5100 Wisconsin Avenue NW, Suite 404, Washington, DC 20016. Phone: (202) 686-2210. Fax: (202) 686-2216.

United Poultry Concerns (UPC), P.O. Box 150, Machipongo, Virginia 23405. Phone: (757) 678-7875.

Vegetarian Resource Group (VRG), P.O. Box 1463, Baltimore, MD 21203. Phone: (410) 366-8343. Fax: (410) 366-8804.

Index